Why bad policy persists:

Examining finance practitioners' views of the English NHS internal market

Dear Julie,

I thought you might want to see a copy of this now it is done! Hope all is well with you. You know where we are. P16 of the magazine gives you a mentu.
All the best and love,
Lee and Deb xx

Why bad policy persists:

Examining finance practitioners' views of the English NHS internal market

First published 2024

This book is copyright. All rights reserved. No part of this publication may be reproduced or distributed in any form or by any means, or stored in a database or retrieval system, without the prior written permission of the author.

© Lee Outhwaite 2024

British Library Cataloguing-in-Publication Data
A catalogue record for this book is available from the British Library

ISBN: 979-8300810-16-0

All the views expressed in this book are the views of the author alone. They do not represent either the views of the Healthcare Financial Management Association (HFMA) or Oxford Value & Stewardship Programme (OVSP) or Liaison Group or Fleet Solutions.

Interior layout and cover design by Bicester Publishing Ltd
www.bicesterpublishing.co.uk

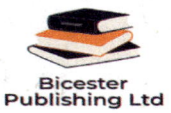

Why bad policy persists:

Examining finance practitioners' views of the English NHS internal market

Lee Outhwaite

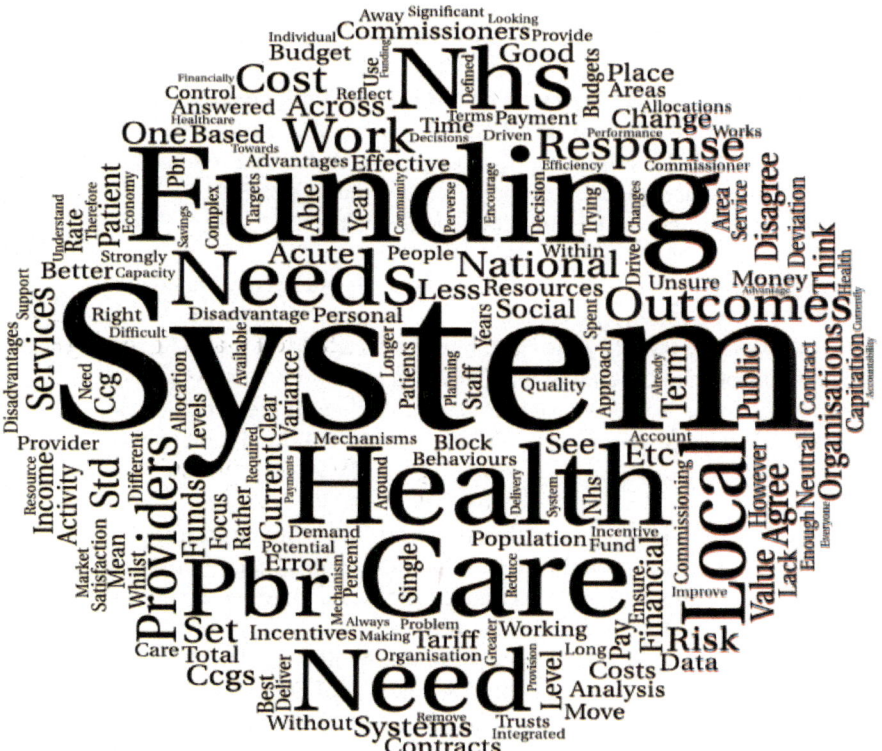

CONTENTS

List of Abbreviations	vii
List of Figures and Tables	ix
Foreward (by Muir Gray)	xiii
Preface	xiv
Acknowledgements	xviii
Abstract	xix

Chapter 1 – Introduction: Key Conceptual Problems and Research Questions — 21
1.1 Context — 21
1.2 Key conceptual problems impacting the research — 23
1.3 The challenge of the internal market — 29
1.4 Research aims and research questions — 32
1.5 Practitioner research and reflective practice — 35

Chapter 2 – Literature Review: The NHS, New Public Management, Quasi-Markets and Policy Implementation — 39
2.1 The English NHS: History, Originating Structure and Development — 39
2.2 New Public Management, Market Challenge and the NHS — 42
2.3 The Development of the Market in the English NHS — 50
2.4 2012 Health Act and Quasi – 'Market 3' — 56
2.5 Assessing the Internal Market and Current Management Arrangements and Views on their Replacement — 59
2.6 Further Accounts of the Reasons for and Frailties of the English NHS Market — 72
2.7 Theories of Public Policy Implementation — 78
2.8 Top Down and Bottom-Up Approaches to Policy Implementation, the Role of Epistemic Groups and the Advocacy Coalition Framework — 83
2.9 Literature Review Conclusions — 88

Chapter 3 – Methodology: Positionality and Practitioner Research — 91
3.1 Practitioner Research and the Evolving Role of this Practitioner — 91
3.2 Selecting Methodologies to Appraise Healthcare Funding, Practitioner Views and Policy Development — 95
3.3 Ethical Considerations and Access to Information and Participants — 97
3.4 Abductive, Action and Practitioner Research and Ongoing Enquiry — 102
3.5 Is NHS Funding Sophisticated Enough to Run a Market? — 107
3.6 What are Finance Practitioners' Attitudes, and have they Impacted on Policy Success? — 110
3.7 Are Finance Practitioners an Epistemic Community Able to Influence Policy? — 118

3.8 Research and Career Overlaps: Biases and Opportunities	118
3.9 Health Policy and Key Analytical Themes within the Study	123

Chapter 4 – Findings: Do Finance Practitioners believe NHS funding could run a market? — 127

4.1 The Nature of English NHS Healthcare Organisation Funding	128
4.2 The Costing and Pricing of NHS Treatment and Care in England	131
4.3 Practitioner Views on English NHS Provider Financial Performance	135
4.4 Bivariate Regression Analysis into causal factors for health provider financial performance 2016/17	140
4.4.1 Financial Performance versus Turnover	140
4.4.2 Financial Performance versus Reference Cost Index	141
4.4.3 Financial Performance versus Reference Cost/Turnover	143
4.4.4 Financial Performance versus Income from main CCG	144
4.4.5 Financial Performance versus CCG Financial Performance	146
4.4.6 Financial Performance versus CCG Distance from Target	147
4.4.7 Financial Performance versus Market Forces Factor	147
4.4.8 Financial Performance versus NHSE Income	148
4.4.9 Financial Performance versus PFI Assets	149
4.4.10 Financial Performance versus Education and Research Income	150
4.4.11 Financial Performance versus CQC Rating and Four-Hour Wait Standard	151
4.4.12 Overall Summary of Financial Performance Regression Work	154
4.5 Multivariate Regression of the Healthcare Provider Funding as a Response to the Action Research	156
4.6 Conclusions from Discussion on Healthcare Provider Funding Analysis	158

Chapter 5 – Findings : What are Finance Practitioner's Views on the Internal Market? — 161

5.1 The Author's Practitioner View on the Internal Market System	161
5.2 The Impact of the Practitioner Views on NHS Market Policy and HFMA/PwC (2018 Report)	165

Chapter 6 - Findings - How do Finance Practitioners Influence Policy? — 189

6.1 The Role of Evidence in the Development of Public Policy	189
6.2 Overview and Role of Action Research	197
6.3 Overview of Findings on Healthcare Funding and Practitioner Views via the HFMA Policy and Research Committee	200
6.4 Summary on the Impact of Evidence and Practitioner Views on NHS Finance and Internal Market Policy	205

Chapter 7 – Conclusions, Recommendations and Proposed Further Research	213
7.1 Do Finance Practitioners believe the way the NHS is funded could run an internal market?	213
7.2 What are finance practitioners' views on the NHS internal market and what have the impact of those views been?	214
7.3 How do Finance Practitioners Influence Policy?	216
7.4 Overall Conclusions	220
7.5 Recommendations	225
7.6 Proposed Further Research	228
References	231

List of Abbreviations

ACF	Advocacy Coalition Framework
A&E	Accident and Emergency Department
APPG	All Party Parliamentary Working Group
BMJ	British Medical Journal
CCG	Clinical Commissioning Groups
CIPFA	Chartered Institute of Finance and Accountancy
CQUIN	Commissioning for Quality and Innovation
CQC	Care Quality Commission
DLUHC	Department of Levelling Up, Housing and Communities
DoH	Department of Health
DHSC	Department of Health and Social Care
ED	Emergency Department
FT	Foundation Trust
GDP	Gross Domestic Product
GP	General Practice
HFMA	Healthcare Financial Management Association
HRG	Healthcare Resource Groups
ICB	Integrated Care Board
ICS	Integrated Care Systems
I&E	Income and Expenditure
MFF	Market Forces Factor

MLR	Multivariate Linear Regression
NHSE	NHS England
NHSI	NHS Improvement
NAO	National Audit Office
NPM	New Public Management
PbR	Payments by Results
PCT	Primary Care Trust
PFI	Private Finance Initiative
PwC	Price Waterhouse Coopers
QuANGO	Quasi-Autonomous Non-Government Organisation
QOF	Quality and Outcomes Framework
RCI	Reference Cost Index
STF	Sustainability and Transformation Funding
STP	Sustainability and Transformation Plans (latterly Partnerships)
TDA	Trust Development Authority
WAU	Weighted Activity Unit
WHO	World Health Organisation

List of Figures and Tables

Word Frequency Cloud Associated with HFMA/PwC practitioner research

Figure 1.1: Triple Value Healthcare – Gray Model

Figure 1.2: What makes and keeps us healthy and well, diagram by Dean Wallace, Director of Public Health, Derbyshire County Council

Figure 1.3: The Health Financial Challenge, designed by the author, for health finance teaching

Figure 2.1: UK Expenditure on Health from Harker (2019)

Figure 2.2: Health Reform in 2005 – Diagrammatic Representation

Figure 2.3: Into the labyrinth: BMJ (2017) UK health and social care funding

Figure 2.4: HFMA - The "current" England 2018 NHS structure and organisations

Figure 3.1: Research Chronology and the Author's Changes in Roles

Figure 3.2: The interrelationship between the three central research approaches

Figure 3.3: Research Chronology, the changing English NHS and Changing Research Design

Figure 4.1: Department of Health (2007) Schematic - Introduction of Payments by Results

Figure 4.2: Author's Own Diagram - Approach to Improvement within the Hospital Setting

Figure 4.3: NAO (2018) Surplus/Deficits of Trusts 2010/11 to 2017/18

Figure 4.4: Deficit position of Trusts 2016/17 compared to 2017/18

Figure 4.5: Regression 1 - Deficit percentage of Trusts 2016/17 compared to Trust turnover.

Figure 4.6: Regression 2 – Deficit percentage of Trusts compared to Reference Cost Index

Figure 4.7: Regression 3 – Deficit percentage compared to Reference Cost Submission Total

Figure 4.8: Regression 4 – Deficit percentage compared to proportion of income from main CCG.

Figure 4.9: The Author's CCG allocation calculation methodology

Figure 4.10: Regression 5 – Deficit percentage of Trusts compared to level of CCG deficit.

Figure 4.11: Regression 6 – Deficit percentage compared to CCG Distance from Target

Figure 4.12: Regression 7 – Deficit percentage compared to Market Forces Factor

Figure 4.13: Regression 8 – Deficit percentage compared to NHSE % income to Trust:

Figure 4.14: Regression 9 – Deficit percentage compared with PFI Assets

Figure 4.15: Regression 10 – Deficit percentage compared with education and research income.

Figure 4.16: Regression 11 – Deficit percentage compared to Care Quality Commission Rating

Figure 4.17: Regression 12 – Deficit Percentage Compared with Four-Hour Performance

Figure 5.1: HFMA/PwC practitioner research coding analysis of Q5. "Is funding fit-for-purpose".

Figure 5.2: HFMA/PwC research coding on "advantages and disadvantages of capitation-based system"

Figure 5.3: HFMA/PwC practitioner research coding analysis of Q11 "outcomes"

Figure 5.4: HFMA/PwC research coding analysis "The NHS is funded and the reforms needed".

Figure 5.5: Summary Schematic of the HFMA/PwC report findings

Figure 6.1: An Original Summary Schematic of the Complex Map of How NHS Policy is Shaped

Figure 5.5: Summary Schematic of the HFMA/PwC report findings

Figure 6.1: An Original Summary Schematic of the Complex Map of How NHS Policy is Shaped

Figure 6.2: Summary Sphere of Influence: Changing the Internal Market - Allies, Opponents and Neutrals (Hart and Bond, 1995)

Figure 6.3: Force Field Analysis Developed by the Author on the Internal Market

Figure 7.1: Politics, Policy, Adoption and Professional Practice in the NHS Internal Market

Table 1.1: Commonwealth Fund Assessment of Care System Performance

Table 2.1: Differences between the 1991 and 2002 market reforms (Ham, 2009: 9)

Table 2.2: A Blueprint to map the current 'market' to a tidied up English NHS (Paton (2016);197)

Table 3.1: The Human Perspective: Methodological Dimensions - Bruyn (1963)

Table 3.2: Attitudinal Research Strategy: Adapted from Bhaskar by Blaikie (2007)

Table 3.3: Matrix of Health Policy and Research Key Analytical Themes

Table 4.1: Regression Analysis Variables on Healthcare Organisation Financial Performance

Table 4.2: Bivariate Regression Summary Healthcare Organisation Financial Performance

Table 5.1: HFMA/PwC research on which funding mechanisms help organisations work together.

Table 5.2: HFMA/PwC research do you understand the financial drivers for your organisation.

Table 5.3: HFMA/PwC research on a move away from the market to integrated care

Table 5.4: HFMA/PwC research on statements about long term funding

Table 5.5: HFMA/PwC practitioner research on statements about outcomes

Table 6.1: 2015, 2017 and 2019 Conservative, Labour and Liberal Democrat Manifesto References to NHS Structural Reform

Table 6.2: Action Research Questionnaire (Hart and Bond (1995))

Table 6.3: Internal Market Policy Success by the time of the 2022 Act, populated by the author, using McConnell's (2010) approach.

FOREWORD

There are two important and inter-related themes in this research, which are both of vital importance to the NHS.

The first is a study of the organisational changes that have been introduced over the years in attempt to manage one of the most complex challenges on earth, meeting the healthcare needs of a population equitably and optimally from a finite resource base. There have been numerous attempts to do this, some based on Acts of Parliament, some on managerial opinion but all failing to produce the desired result. His conclusion is that the most recent Act offers some hope because it brings together the two main options, markets and bureaucracies because "the 2022 Act does not abolish the internal market, but incorporates more place-based structures alongside it". The names of the organisations are also welcome with the word System prominent reflecting Oliver Williamson's principles that some challenges are too complex to be solved by either markets or bureaucracies and need systems.

The second theme is a study, which could be classified as anthropological, of the community of finance professionals and their contribution to achieving not only optimal outcome but also the very survival of the NHS. He defines the need to recognise that finance professionals need to be recognised as an 'epistemic' community, a network with skills and knowledge with a vitally but under-appreciated contribution to make to the survival of the NHS. He concludes that this community of finance professionals "should propose more integrated working and policies that focus on population health and closer ties with local government to ensure an integrated system works more effectively, to deliver a higher value health and care system."

This thesis is a call to arms for finance professionals, too often seen as, and seeing themselves as, passive implementers of policy to be become leaders and the role of leadership is to change culture to a culture which focuses on value as well as efficiency.

It is very well written, and very timely.

Muir Gray

The Oxford Value and Stewardship Programme (OVSP)

PREFACE

With various leaves of absence, and the pandemic I have spent over 14 years (very on and off) studying for and writing my doctoral thesis, which is the document you see before you. The original motivation for the doctorate surrounded the idea of evidence-based management and public policy; and a growing belief that the NHS internal market didn't really add much value. What follows this preface is the doctorate in full, with the appendices removed. I have left it as an academic monograph to provide an example of what Level 8 study looks like for those other colleagues in NHS finance who may have a doctoral thesis in them. In my view, we need more practitioner research in healthcare finance. I wasn't intending to publish the document, however, I was persuaded to, by Muir Gray, so here it is; to coincide with my HFMA Presidential Year.

Since the submission of the doctorate and the associated minor amendments much has happened, not least the election of the new Labour government. It will be interesting to see what policy course is now taken in the interests of "mission-based government" and how we manage the public sector beyond the silos in which it has been traditionally managed. It really feels like it is time for a new public policy management paradigm to emerge beyond the "new public management" approach of targets and markets. There is the need for a description of the positive impact of the assertive role for the state and the assertive role for the public finance accountant. This new approach needs to empower frontline staff in a very different way - around the broader and hugely complex work which we all try to do - trying to make citizens lives fairer, more equal, and more inclusive. In my view, a very good start in this thinking is represented by a recent Demos paper, 'Liberated Public Services: A New Vision for Citizens, Professionals and Policy Makers'.[1]

The 14 years when I have been under-taking this work has also been the period of worsening NHS performance which has also been the period in which the NHS has seen the lowest growth rates in funding it has experienced since its formation. This position is very well described in The Rise and Decline of the NHS in England by Ham.[2] There is a difficulty in concluding whether there is a need for changing how the service operates and is structured, and the need for a more robust funding approach. The honest answer is probably both are needed but there is then a paradox around the lack of appetite for another top-down re-organisation and the potential need for one in terms the wider integration

---

[1] Glover B. (2024) Liberated Public Services: A New Vision for Citizens, Professionals and Policy Makers London: Demos

[2] Ham C. (2023) The Rise and Decline of the NHS in England: How political failure led to the crisis in the NHS and Social Care London: Kings Fund

and prevention and anticipatory care agendas. The need for a more open and honest conversation about the required funding is also addressed in a more recent paper by Appleby, Leng and Marshall, NHS funding for a secure future, which recommends continued funding through taxation, an independent office of NHS budgetary responsibility, longer terms planning and an immediate cash injection to start to recover the £32bn shortfall in funding from 2010 to 2020.[3]

Despite the potential funding shortfall, there is a need in health for a much better approach to value based healthcare and a need to assess the efficient operation of health and care services much more widely. This will require a different approach beyond that which was used in the internal market. This new approach will focus on population health management and truly addresses the challenge of socially determined disease. The work of Marmot, Gray and Mintzberg are all important in defining the need for and signalling a change in approach. The healthcare system is broken, but it perhaps isn't the participants in the system that have broken it. It has been a reluctance to really trying to integrate beyond the structures we currently inhabit.

The brokenness of the system is outlined in a relatively recent book by Dorling, Shattered Nation.[4] Here Dorling describes how modern Britain has become more and more unequal and he notes a redefinition of the Beveridge five giants Want, Disease, Ignorance, Squalor and Idleness, (following the Second World War) with their updated version Hunger, Precarity, Waste, Exploitation, and Fear (in the UK of today). The book left me wondering about the extent to which we could really offer a free at the point of need universal healthcare system with a society this unequal. Sobering and worrying stuff. Challenging inequality has to be a first priority.

The need for a renewal of the role of the state is then further outlined in the recent book by Hutton, This Time No Mistakes.[5] Here Hutton describes how we need to escape some of the grip of the UKs adherence to laissez-faire economics to develop a truly efficient state. He suggests twelve key areas for action on how to improve the UK polity, noting how much room for improvement there is in each of these areas. For the public finance accountant he also makes some important recommendations on the need for enhanced levels of public investment through rejuvenated public institutions.

Over the last 14 years particularly, but not exclusively, it would seem like there have been various episodes of poor policy solutions which have not therefore

---

3 Appleby J., Leng G. and Marshall M. (2024) NHS funding for a secure future London: BMJ 20/3/24
4 Dorling D. (2023) Shattered Nation: Inequality and the Geography of A Failing State London: Verso
5 Hutton W. (2024) This Time No Mistakes: How to Remake Britain London: Head of Zeus

had a really deep understanding of systems thinking, in my own area of health. I am not personally persuaded that the problem of ambulances queueing at hospitals is solved by putting more ambulances on the road. I am not persuaded that specific targets around recruiting health visitors (in a shorter period of time that they can be trained) doesn't have an unintended consequence on the midwifery workforce (it caused some of them to retrain and left us a void!). I am not sure that policy approaches around virtual wards or the additional role reimbursement scheme don't have unintended consequences, unless implemented well and owned differently at a local level. We need a different regionalism and localism in our public policy towards health, healthcare and broader well-being.

I am increasingly interested in an approach to undefended leadership and all staff being associated with improving their work that builds on the Toyota Production System and the Virginia Mason production system. It would seem that the work in Leeds and Coventry Hospitals (on the Leeds Way and UHCWi approaches, respectively) are beginning to liberate frontline staff to improve the work they do themselves. There is a need for a strong quality improvement methodology and an approach in the public sector which we all need to galvanise around to deliver service change. The accountancy profession in the public sector, beyond the introduction of artificial intelligence, will probably need to embrace a new role around quality improvement, the understanding of waste, value stream mapping and building improvement capability.

The NHS impact framework around building shared vision and purpose, investing in people and culture, developing the right leadership behaviours, an approach to improvement capability and capacity and the need for embedding improvement in our management system and processes seems like a really good start on this journey. Over the next five years, we'll see a very different approach to delivering health care, which will be far more personalised, predictive and needs to be for more integrated with other parts of the public services. We will need to be able to implement technological change far more rapidly to ensure value for both our health and care (and wider) public sector workforce and our public. We will need a better community, and society engagement in that mission and perhaps it is time to revisit, through a new NHS commission how we will deliver a healthcare system for the future.

Within NHS finance, this will give us some specific work to do working with other agencies and other professions, there will be a need for a health and care production system, perhaps one that moves into local government more fully, and also into education, housing, work and pensions and the criminal justice system to really deliver more effective integrated services. We will need to work beyond the silos which we have traditionally operated in to deliver this approach.

We will need to have better measures of high value health care which rise above reducing costs of some of our old production currencies. The costs of socially determined disease are exceptionally high. We will need a new finance regime for high value health care, and we will need to be a lot better at costing for waste and costing for value to enable us to carry on delivering the NHS and wider public services in a truly more economic, efficient, and effective way.

Lee Outhwaite

November 2024

ACKNOWLEDGEMENTS

I would like to thank all those that participated in the research undertaken as part of this project. Without the responses to the requests for data, the wider questionnaire work, the willingness of the HFMA and HFMA Policy and Research Committee to help; and all the many inspiring NHS colleagues I have worked with in my career, this work would not have been possible. I'd like to thank Paul Baumann, the former Director of Finance at NHS England; and Bob Alexander, the former Director of Finance at NHS Improvement; for their help and support, and for consenting to give access to much of the financial data. I'd also like to thank, the HFMA/PwC research stakeholder group, who were always exceptionally well-informed on health, policy, and government. Also, thanks to David Morris and Emma Knowles (PwC and HFMA, respectively) for granting access to the data described in Chapter 5. And thanks to Ian Moston and Mark Knight (former HFMA Policy and Research Chair and HFMA CEO,) for granting access to the HFMA Policy and Research Subcommittee which acted as the main group to pursue the action research phase of the project.

Also, thanks to Philip Catney, (particularly), and also Calum Paton, Dana Rosenfeld, Ronnie Lippens and Steve Cropper, at the University of Keele, for their help in instilling the thesis with an element of academic rigour, and many other contributions, at various stages. Many thanks to Mark Wickham-Jones, particularly, at the University of Bristol, who taught me about the New Right and Public Choice, and patiently supervised my undergraduate dissertation on the privatisation of British Coal. I have also now read his book (1986) "Economic Strategy and the Labour Party: Politics and Policy-Making 1970 to 1983". I should have read it sooner. My degree at the University of Bristol set me off thinking about new public management. There are links between my thinking around the imperfect privatisation of electricity and coal in the 1980s, which was discussed in my undergraduate dissertation, and thinking which is contained in this thesis around the nature of the NHS internal market.

Thanks to my Mum and Dad, Geraldine, and David, for all their help and support. Also, Bob Puttock, my father-in-law, gave a near-final draft a very thorough proofread, thank you. Lastly, apologies to my wife, Deborah, and my children, Elizabeth, Joanna, and William, for the time I have spent working on this when really I should have been with them. I'd also like to thank Deborah, further, for all her proofreading assistance, wider advice, and her love. Even, if the resultant document is poor in places or throughout, it would have been a good deal poorer without their help and understanding.

ABSTRACT

This thesis evaluates the reasons for the longevity of the English NHS internal market policy, which challenged the post-1948 public provision model for healthcare services. It reviews the intellectual underpinning of the policy, derived from New Public Management thinking, and describes phases in the evolution of the NHS internal market: "Working for Patients" (1989); "Creating a Patient Led NHS" (2005); and then the 2012 Health and Social Care Act. The policy had considerable longevity considering the various calls and moves to supersede elements of the internal market and replace it. These calls have led to the English Health and Care Act (2022) which seeks to enable healthcare (and wider partner) organisations to work together more easily, but does not abolish the internal market, but incorporates more place-based structures alongside it.

The research examines the views of the epistemic finance practitioner groups involved in administering the NHS internal market, along with the reflective and reflexive practice of the author who has worked in senior roles in NHS finance since 1993. The funding approach for English NHS provider organisations is discussed via quantitative research with fellow practitioners. This research suggests that practitioners do not believe the general approach, or the funding mechanisms were sufficiently robust to run a market.

The thesis then reviews senior finance practitioners' views on the internal market policy itself using questionnaire-based research with a wide sample of NHS finance practitioners. The research assesses the extent of support for the internal market policy and views on its reform. Access to practitioner networks was made possible via the author's positions within the Healthcare Finance Management Association (HFMA) and the Chartered Institute of Public Finance and Accountancy (CIPFA). The research assesses the extent to which the bottom-up views of practitioners may have influenced policy.

The research then moves on to addressing the nature of the use of evidence for public policy formulation and adoption. This action research phase explores the appetite of practitioners to influence English healthcare finance and NHS system management. It suggests reasons why the market approach to the NHS survived for so long and suggests why there was indecision on what should replace it. It concludes that despite the changes introduced in the 2022 Act, there are improvements to NHS finance and structures that could be made and that English NHS finance practitioners should have a policy determination and implementation role. It suggests finance practitioners, as an epistemic community, should propose more integrated working and policies that focus on population health and closer ties with local government to ensure an integrated system works more effectively, to deliver a higher value health and care system.

CHAPTER 1

Introduction: key conceptual problems and research questions

1.1 Context

This professional doctorate is, to a large extent, the product of the author's now thirty-year career in NHS finance. During this time, the NHS in England has had an internal market in health which has separated the commissioning (planning and purchasing) from the provision (delivery and production) of healthcare services. The English NHS is currently going through another reorganisation to try and create a more coherent and integrated set of structures following the passage of the Health and Social Care Act (2022), though some of the key assumptions of the internal market remain. The Bill preceding the Act was described by the Nuffield Trust (2021: 2) as:

> The Bill will overwrite the current local structure of the NHS, where local Clinical Commissioning Groups pay NHS trusts and others to provide care in what is meant to be a competitive "internal market". Instead, under clauses 12 to 25 of the Bill, representatives of trusts, GPs and councils will sit together on the boards of "Integrated Care Systems" (ICSs) responsible for overseeing health services in 42 regions. Each of these will also have a wider partnership committee making plans for greater cooperation across health and social care.

This is not the first attempt to try and improve the management and approaches of the NHS (see Chapter 2). A previous attempt to reorganise the NHS led to a British Medical Journal (BMJ) editorial by Smith et al. (2001: 1) which noted:

> The NHS does not need a distracting and unproved reorganisation that, for all the rhetoric about devolution, leaves unchanged, or even strengthened, the capacity for the centre to micromanage the service into the ground. What is required is a fundamental rethinking of the relationship between central government and the NHS.

There is a tension between the stated aims of the 2022 Act and the reality of policy implementation and intent. The thesis is, therefore, timely in the context of this latest management change for the English NHS, which will have many impacts. One of the immediate impacts resulted in the author taking up a new post in the revised structure, created by the Health and Care Act (2022), as the Chief Financial Officer of the South Yorkshire Integrated Care

Board. The author hence both commentates on and participates in the system through his role as a Director of Finance, via his role as a Trustee of the Healthcare Financial Management Association (HFMA), and via his serving on the Chartered Institute of Public Finance and Accountancy (CIPFA) Council. The thesis, therefore, is steeped in the understanding (and potential agency) the author has. This is not just a desk-top review of health policy; it is based on the participation and access of the author to the NHS system and how he and his colleagues have experienced that policy.

In this thesis, the author asserts that the Health and Care Act (2022) is an important and necessary move away from the internal market, but, in the end, it is concluded that the persistence of the policy's key ideas and policy legacies remain significant challenges to the new structures. The extent to which the internal market policy was in place within the English NHS for longer than the evidence for its efficacy should have allowed has been the subject of much comment. A key reason for this persistence in the face of counterargument and evidence is the idea of "path dependency". Kay (2005: 558) described:

> Path dependency is an appealing concept for understanding public policy development; it provides a label for the empirical observations and intuitions that policies, once established, can be difficult to change or reform.

Path dependence is associated with suboptimal policies enduring for longer than they can be justified (Pierson, 2000; Greener, 2002; Torfing, 2009). There are numerous explanations as to why certain policies endure, particularly in relation to health policy (Saldin, 2017). These can include problems with how political institutions approach policymaking, including in terms of partisanship (Hicks, 2013; Saldin, 2017), and the role of interest groups (Greener, 2005) which seek to maintain the existing policy settlement. [6]

The author subscribes to the view that the NHS internal market and pre-existing structures were suboptimal, but the 2022 Act seems to demonstrate that policy makers and participants seem to believe the English NHS and its systems are only capable of being reviewed and rebuilt from the status quo, incrementally[7]. The 2022 Act does not, the author contends, go far enough and he is keen to see whether the view of a need for greater change is shared by his colleagues.

---

[6] Explaining how and why change occurs in the face of such forces has been a key part of health policy analysis (see Haeder, 2012 and for a challenge to the idea of path dependency in the NHS, see Ross 2007).

[7] The nature of the evolving market in the English NHS is described in Chapter 2, and the ideas of path dependency and policy persistence are revisited in Chapter 7.

The thesis is hence interested in why the epistemic community – which he is a part of in NHS Finance – did not promote more creative ways to abandon and overhaul the internal market policy, which is central to the idea of policy persistence. As Coate and Morris (1999: 1) noted:

> Conventional wisdom in political economy warns that once an economic policy is introduced, it is likely to persist. Even when its original rationale is no longer applicable or has been proven invalid, a policy will prove hard to remove.

The thesis argues that a similar pattern occurred with the NHS internal market. It was a policy that was established from a particular set of ideological rationales, and the policy persisted beyond the point at which the clear limitations of the policy were hard to ignore. Practitioners, as part of broader epistemic communities, play a key in providing and interpreting evidence of problems in policy systems and feeding that back to higher levels of the policy system. They are hence a potentially critically important set of actors in explaining policy continuity and change. Exploring the role of finance professionals in the NHS internal market is important to ascertain the extent to which these practitioners exercised this role around policy change and what barriers they may have experienced to playing this feedback role to help elicit that change.

1.2 Key Conceptual Problems Impacting the Research

How a practitioner influences and tries to improve the system in which they operate is the key focus of this research. This theme is explored in the context of the English healthcare system. A key conceptual challenge for this research is the issue of determining how well a healthcare system is operating, or whether how it is organised is adding value. Such assessments are difficult and fraught with conceptual and methodological challenges. With these challenges in mind, the author is keen to understand how the NHS internal market has or has not helped to improve the operation of the service. To this end, there are three key problems which challenge the analysis of the system in place that the author considers important: 1) assessing the principal policy aims of the English NHS and then consequently the cause and effect associated with public policy interventions; 2) defining value in healthcare and how that can be measured; and 3) addressing the broader social determinants of disease, and the extent to which the English NHS is set up to address these broader issues and/or should be. These three conceptual problems are explored further in the literature review (Chapter 2).

The internal market in the English NHS, introduced in 1989 and still in situ despite the 2022 Act, separates the roles of commissioners and providers in the

NHS. There is, therefore, a separation between those organisations who purchase healthcare services for their allotted populations, and those organisations who provide those healthcare services. There is also an institutional separation between health and social care, which is reflected in Whitehall: health is administered by the Department of Health and Social Care (DHSC) while social care is administered by the Department for Levelling Up, Housing and Communities (DLUHC), via upper tier authorities in local government. DHSC is responsible for the management of the NHS, whereas DLUHC is responsible for managing local government. Local government delivers local policies to deliver public health and broader health and well-being. The name of the Department of Health (DoH) was changed in 2018 to the Department of Health and Social Care, but social services are still predominantly run, and funded separately, through local government. Therefore, there are two potential fractures in policy delivery. Firstly, the purchaser/provider split in the NHS, and secondly, the historic separation between the DHSC and DLUHC. The difficulties of the purchaser/provider split in health are described extensively in what comes in this thesis. Furthermore, the divide between local actors who deliver NHS services within the DHSC, and the services which more broadly contribute to the determinants of health managed by DLUHC are also described.[8]

When assessing the impact of health public policy, particularly concerning the English NHS, it is important to know how policy goals for the service are set, established, and then monitored and evaluated. The overall policies associated with the NHS as a whole can be assessed individually or severally through different objectives such as i) the measurement of the efficiency of the service, ii) the equity of access to services, iii) the equity of outcomes related to particular diseases, or iv) the total average life expectancy for the whole population, or v) the comparative healthy life expectancies of the wealthiest and poorest elements of the population. The goals are, therefore, multiple and evaluation of performance in a complex system such as the NHS is challenging. As a large, bureaucratic, socially embedded structure it is perhaps unsurprising that there is a lack of absolute clarity as to what precisely are the policy goals of the English NHS. There are targets for emergency and elective waiting times, but there is little to determine what the broader success measures of the NHS should be. For example, should they be i) to run the most efficient service, ii) to ensure that there is the most equitable access to services, or iii) to have the best-targeted interventions (e.g. cancer survival rates), or iv) to have a broader, general set of outcomes (e.g. the highest average age of death) as a nation, or v) to close health outcome inequalities between richest and poorest (e.g. the differences between healthy life expectancy). If the NHS is trying to deliver all these objectives, how

---

[8] In addition, these issues are explored in a blog by the author.

is it effectively prioritising between them? An effective funding system is a key input in achieving such outcomes and balancing these (Berger and Messer, 2002; McLoughlin and Leatherman, 2003, Tuohy et al., 2004).

An assessment of the relative performance of healthcare services[9] has been conducted by the Commonwealth Fund (cited by Papanicolas and Smith, 2003). This study attempts to look at the "Healthcare Systems Finance and Coverage" and the approaches to running different healthcare systems across the world and tries to identify "common outcome measures" to assess system performance against them. These results are complex and contested but are converted into the relative performance in rank order in five domains. The results seemingly show the UK system in a relatively favourable light. In 2017 the UK was ranked first, (the previous time the approach was undertaken) and in 2021 fourth. It is worth noting that by 2021 the UK ninth out of ten in the context of outcomes, however. The summary of the results of this work by Schneider, Shah, Doty, Tikkanen, Fields, Williams (2021) are shown in Table 1.1, below:

Table 1.1: Commonwealth Fund Assessment of Care System Performance

	AUS	CAN	FRA	GER	NETH	NZ	NOR	SWE	SWIZ	UK	US
OVERALL RANKING	3	10	8	5	2	6	1	7	9	4	11
Access to Care	8	9	7	3	1	5	2	6	10	4	11
Care Process	6	4	10	9	3	1	8	11	7	5	2
Administrative Efficiency	2	7	6	9	8	3	1	5	10	4	11
Equity	1	10	7	2	5	9	8	6	3	4	11
Health Care Outcomes	1	10	6	7	4	8	2	5	3	9	11

Data: Commonwealth Fund analysis.

The Commonwealth Fund assessment of a healthcare system, using (access to care, care process approach, efficiency, equity, and outcomes) is contestable, but this may be a useful framework for thinking about different dimensions of healthcare value. To fully appraise the success of health policy or health policy measures it does require us to determine what we find valuable, and it also means we need to measure and evaluate those things, to determine success.

---

9 The parameters of a 'healthcare system' varies across states, including whether the 'healthcare system' includes the bodies that deliver care such as general practice and hospitals, or includes adult social care, or all the agencies and factors that can contribute to broader health and wellbeing. In addition, there have been attempts to assess the contrasting approaches and outcomes of these systems in comparative public policy (see Papanicolas and Smith, 2013: 33).

How different healthcare system goals and priorities are managed, described, and monitored is contentious and difficult. The latest strategic refresh for the English NHS is The NHS Long-Term Plan (2019). This document has stated aims for new service models, more prevention, the tackling of health inequalities, and setting standards for improvements in specific areas of care. It notes an approach to address the workforce pressures the service is under and advises on the further use of technology and notes an improved funding settlement. It also called for the NHS and wider partners to work in a more integrated way, and it also called for primary legislation to support the acceleration of this integration, which it was thought would lead to more optimal care. The purchaser/provider split in the NHS has given rise to several different provider organisations, which are called upon to work more closely together in a more integrated way.

> . . . . the NHS and our partners will be moving to create Integrated Care Systems everywhere by April 2021, building on the progress already made. ICSs bring together local organisations in a pragmatic and practical way to deliver the 'triple integration' of primary and specialist care, physical and mental health services, and health with social care. They will have a key role in working with Local Authorities at 'place' level, and through ICSs, commissioners will make shared decisions with providers on population health, service redesign and Long-Term Plan implementation. (The NHS Long Term Plan, 2019: 10).

This thesis is interested in the broader definitions of the value of the systems and the services offered. Gray (2017) has identified different layers of measuring value in healthcare, which is shown in Figure 1.1. Firstly, Gray identifies productivity and the need to drive down the costs of the delivery of healthcare outputs. Next, Gray identifies the cost of outcomes to define the next layer of efficiency. Further, he identifies the need to ensure we are utilising services well and not over or under-treating patients, and finally, he identifies the need to ensure that patients and citizens receive services that they find value-adding. This, he states, gives rise to technical, allocative, and personal value. Gray describes the delivery of all these levels of efficiency of value as "triple value healthcare".

Figure 1.1: Triple Value Healthcare – Gray Model

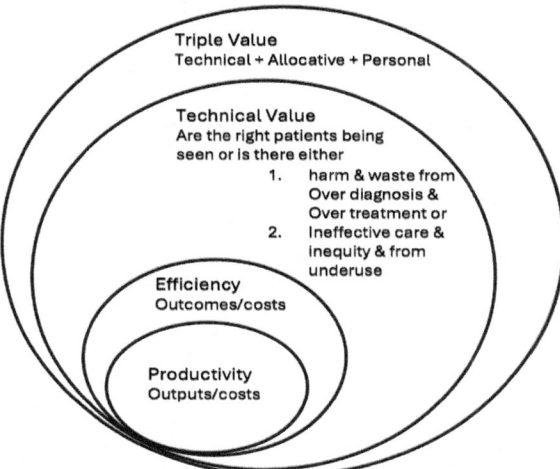

This thesis asserts that the internal market in health has made the provider organisations concentrate mainly on productivity, whilst commissioning and local government have tried to champion the wider value of healthcare. However, this separation may not have led to services being delivered optimally. Also, the separation between health and well-being, amplified by the separation between the DHSC and the NHS on the one hand, and the DLUHC and local government bodies on the other hand, may have contributed to this lack of optimum delivery.

Health, therefore, can be viewed very broadly and can include personal reflections on the value individuals personally receive and experience from healthcare, or the view of the success of the health system can focus on productivity and a much narrower view of efficiency. The author is more minded in his approach to take this broader view of triple value healthcare when answering the question of the value of a system or in potentially determining the nature of the impact which the policy of an internal market has had.

Healthcare delivery viewed more broadly involves looking at the health of the population and what fundamentally causes ill health. The Marmot Review (2010) looked at the broader determinants of health and made a series of recommendations about how inequity in healthcare outcomes could be addressed. These measures included recommendations in six domains: i) give every child the best start in life, ii) enable all children young people and adults to maximise their capabilities, iii) create fair employment and good work for all, iv) ensure a healthy standard of living for all, v) create and develop healthy and sustainable places and communities, and, vi) strengthen the role and impact of ill health prevention. Although practically all the recommendations from the review were accepted by the then Coalition Government, the reappraisal of these issues, by Marmot et al (2020) led to some stark conclusions.

> From the beginning of the 20th century, England experienced continuous improvements in life expectancy but from 2011 these improvements slowed dramatically, almost grinding to a halt. For part of the decade 2010-2020 life expectancy actually fell in the most deprived communities, outside London, for women and in some regions for men. For men and women everywhere, the time spent in poor health is increasing...Put simply, if health has stropped improving it is a sign that society has stopped improving. (Marmot et al., 2020: 5).

Research into the precise causes of disease and ill health shows that the contribution of the healthcare service itself, in terms of quality and access to care, is a relatively low contributing factor at around 20% of overall health and well-being. The wider causes of ill health are related to health behaviours, socio-economic factors, and the wider environment. This is shown in Figure 1.2. The Robert Wood Johnson Foundation (which is part of the School of Public Health at Harvard University) research by McGovern et al. (2014: 8) concluded:

> With the increasing appreciation of health as the product of more than access to the health care system and individual behaviours, along with the many opportunities afforded by the Affordable Care Act, comes the chance to transform how we think about health and how we can improve it for the population as a whole.

The author, in his NHS career and through this research, is therefore interested in whether the internal market structure made the NHS think too narrowly about how to improve health and the determinants of health, further demonstrating the problems created by path dependency and policy persistence. The Marmot Review notes the widening gaps between health for different socio-economic groups but does not recommend structural changes within health and care to address this issue. This thesis is keen to understand whether our system of healthcare is as good as the Commonwealth Fund suggested. He also wishes to explore more broadly how the NHS embraces an approach to population health management, and public health and how the NHS works more closely with local government and other branches of Government to deliver improved health outcomes. The thesis explores how population health management and appropriate approaches to improving public health operate in the shadow of the internal market. Also, the author is interested in outcomes being more broadly defined, delivering "triple value healthcare", in keeping with the aims of The NHS Long Term Plan, which challenge and address the broader determinants of health (which are much wider than the clinical care the individual receives). He is also interested in whether the internal market may have hindered these broader aims. The next section of the introduction gives a brief introduction to the internal market and how it is being challenged.

Figure 1.2: What makes and keeps us healthy and well, diagram by Dean Wallace, Director of Public Health, Derbyshire County Council

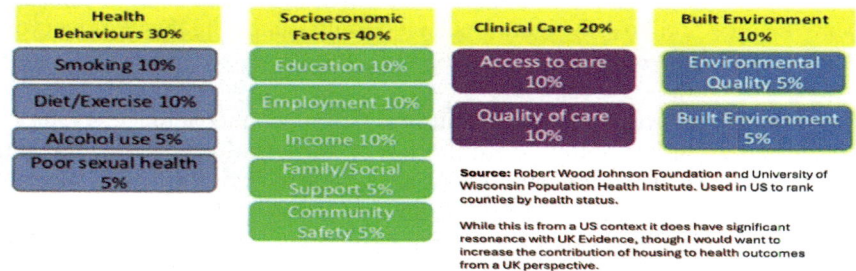

1.3 The Challenge to the Internal Market

An internal market – creating a split between commissioning and provision organisations – in healthcare in the English NHS was introduced via the Department of Health (1989) "Working for Patients" White Paper. It stated that the goal of the internal market should be:

> To enable hospitals which best meet the needs and wishes of their patients to get money to do so, the money required to treat patients will be able to cross administrative boundaries. All hospitals, whether run by health authorities or self-governing will be free to offer their services to different health authorities and to the private sector. (Department of Health, 1989: 5)

At this point, one could question the nature of health and well-being and the extent to which healthcare services, and more particularly hospital services can effectively be separated from primary, community and wider services to the extent that this proposal was and remains sensible. But despite that, since 1989, there has been a continued attempt to run the English NHS through an internal market mechanism, and although the precise reasons for the introduction of that internal market are contested, there has been a continued split in responsibilities between commissioning organisations and those involved with providing NHS services. But policy has been evolving and the structure of the NHS has been rethought and changed since 1989.

The potential frailty of the market mechanism, and the need to evaluate the evidence for the internal market policy, along with the potential ability of the author to influence the system in which he works, have been the reasons for his undertaking this study. The author has adopted the role of a researcher on the internal market, whilst also being a practitioner within that system. This dual role has presented challenges but has also afforded the author a high degree of access to the system and its participants. The study through practitioner research and action research, seeks to explain the fading role of the NHS internal market, at a time when there is a partial legislative attempt to dismantle it. It also seeks to describe why and how the author is trying to influence the development of a replacement for that market.

Some of the originating academic literature and the accounts of the development of the internal market policy are important to this study. The broader aims of the economics of markets are also interwoven with a political standpoint on the role of the state to effectively deliver public policy objectives. The wider positioning of markets to deliver public policy has also been described, evaluated, and sometimes proposed by Le Grand (1991):

> When the Thatcher government came into power in 1979, the welfare state was the biggest area of non-market activity in the British economy...The National Health Service, for example, was the largest employer in Western Europe; and the welfare state as a whole consumed almost a quarter of the Gross Domestic Product...A major offensive against the bureaucratic structure of welfare provision was launched in 1988 and 1989; years that in retrospect will be seen as critical in the history of British social policy. For it was then that the Conservative government began to apply a programme of market-orientated change to the welfare state. (Le Grand, 1991: 1256)

Prior to the development of the internal market, the structures of the NHS were not perfect and there were several accounts of the need for change which are described in Chapter 2. At this point, a key policy decision was being made with advocates for the approach of an internal market and quite strong contrary positions made. The view of Le Grand (1991) at the time was seemingly ambivalent, despite being often cited as a proponent:

> Properly monitored, they [markets in public policy] should be able to provide economists and other analysts of social policy with evidence as to whether, suitably adapted and expanded, quasi-markets

constitute the way forward for social policy - or whether they are a retrograde development that will need reversing as soon as politically or practically feasible. (Le Grand, 1991: 1267).

Whether "they" are and should now be reversed is at issue in this thesis. Another commentator around the advent of the internal market who is often cited is Enthoven, Professor of Public and Private Management at Stanford. He made recommendations on the development of an internal market in health, but perhaps interestingly came up with a model of competing Healthcare Maintenance Organisations (HMOs) – which include primary and secondary care clinicians. Although he is often cited as an early proponent of the market currently in place, it could be contended that the one which was developed and is now in place is not the one which he recommended. Enthoven (1985:13) noted:

> In fact, the structure of the NHS contains perverse incentives. For example, a district that develops an excellent service in some speciality that attracts more referrals is likely to get more work without getting more resources to do it. The district that does a poor job will 'export' patients and have less work, but not correspondingly less resource, for its reward.

The resultant approach of the English NHS to the internal market did correct for this specific perverse incentive, with the money following the patient. However, it could be said that the market that was put in place worsened the divisions between primary and secondary care Enthoven (1985) also observed:

> The NHS appears locked forever into a model with separation between GPs and hospital by specialists. I was told they communicate with each other mostly by mail. In the United States, at least some observers, myself included find there is much to recommend in the multi-specialty group practice in which the primary care physicians are partners in regular contact with specialists, sharing the same offices, records, and equipment. (Enthoven, 1985: 46)

> However, if British policymakers were to examine seriously a radically different scheme for health care, I would recommend the competing HMO model as the most promising candidate. (Enthoven 1985: 49)

The internal market which was introduced in 1989 did seek to address the initial failure identified by Enthoven, related to poor reimbursement for out-of-district care. The internal market which has been in place since then has done little, or perhaps made worse, the close working of the GPs and hospital specialists. The changes proposed in the Long-Term Plan are seeking to address this, and the Healthcare Management Organisations (HMOs) described by Enthoven could be seen as similar to the proposals for Integrated Care Partnerships or Integrated Care Providers, within Integrated Care Systems, that are now being discussed and developed.

1.4 Research Aims and Research Questions

The purpose of this research into the English NHS internal market addresses three aims and objectives and three research questions (RQs):

- Aim 1: to understand the intention and effectiveness of the policy, which created that market environment.
- Aim 2: to assess how views on the policy have impacted on the potential for policy implementation success and persistence.
- Aim 3: to reveal the nature of and extent to which financial practitioners act collectively on policy development and implementation.
- RQ 1: Do finance practitioners believe the way in which the NHS is funded could run a market?
- RQ 2: Have the views of finance practitioners on the internal market impacted policy success and policy persistence?
- RQ 3: To what extent do finance practitioners inside the NHS constitute an epistemic community which is able to influence the development of policy and advocate a move away from the internal market?

Quasi-markets in the English NHS may have been seen as an answer to the fundamental problem of the affordability of the NHS. However, the author believes the quasi-market policy has not effectively addressed this challenge. The aims and research questions seek to understand at a conceptual, delivery and policy advocacy and influence level, how the views of finance practitioners may have influenced the policy success and the changes to the English NHS which are now proposed.

The extent to which the NHS is affordable does impact the scope of its services. Some of the key challenges which the NHS has been dealing with since its inception have been: (i) how it should be organised; (ii) whether is it affordable, and consequently (iii) what the precise scope of the NHS should be. This thesis predominantly explores question the first question, since the author is interested in trying to resolve how the NHS could be better organised, but the thesis contributes to the latter two. These are interrelated issues though, as shown in Figure 1.3 (developed by the author for teaching NHS finance).

There are also the key conceptual problems impacting the research, described above, running through this challenge, around the extent to which there is a) clarity of the policy goals and how the system success for the English NHS is measured, the extent to which there is b) the right definition of healthcare value and c) how the NHS is appropriately addressing the broader causes of ill health.

Although the costs of healthcare systems (and the NHS) described in Figure 1.3, are determined both by the needs of the population and changes in technology, they are also determined by the adequacy of the funding allocation mechanism, how risks are managed within the system, how services are delivered, and the scope of the role of the state. These then feedback to the initial question of whether the system is funded adequately. The purpose of this thesis is to examine the extent to which a quasi-market, with a split between provider and commissioning organisations, is alleviating the financial problems or adding to them.

Figure 1.3: The Health The Health Financial Challenge, designed by the author, for health finance teaching.

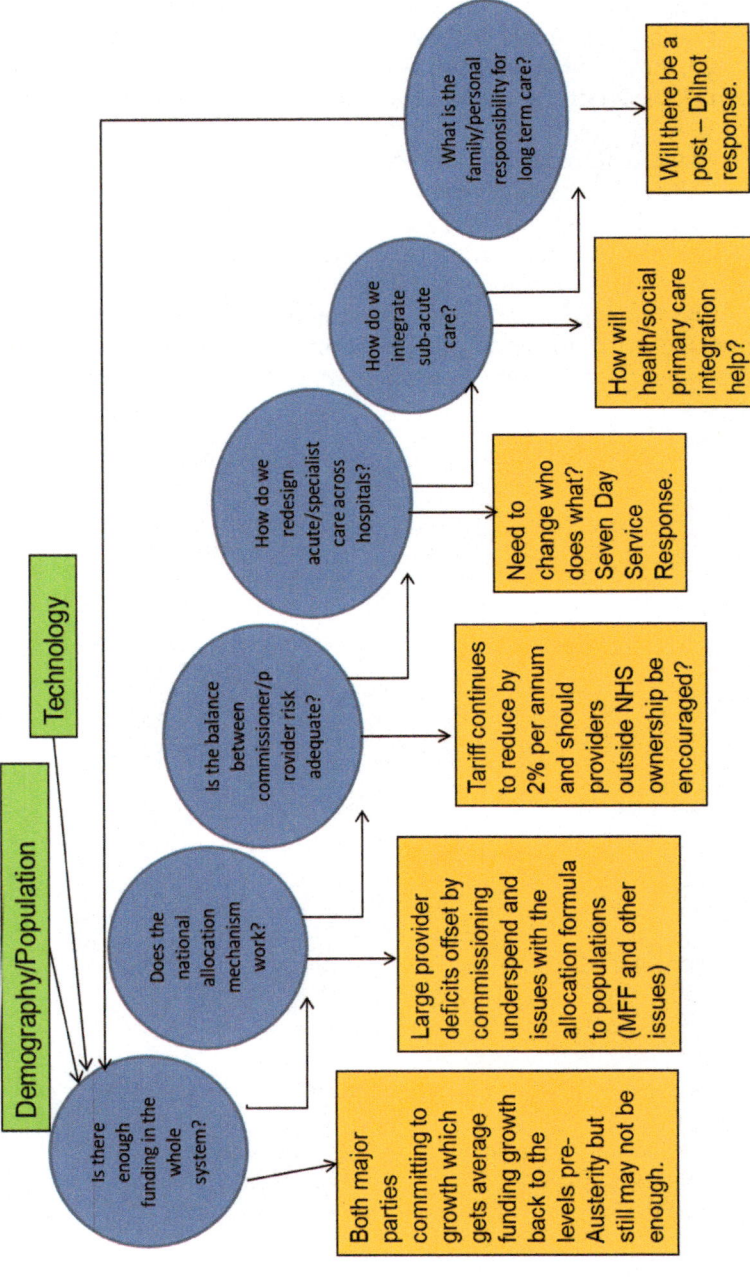

There are fundamental questions to be addressed, beyond the initial funding question, described in Figure 1.3, including the way money is nationally allocated, and how the services are organised, particularly how care integration is best delivered and the role of the state for long-term care, which inform the answer to the primary funding question, and these themes are discussed in this thesis.

1.5 Practitioner Research and Reflective and Reflexive Practice

Whilst undertaking his substantive roles in NHS finance, the author has also worked more widely nationally, via being a Trustee and sitting on, then chairing, the Policy and Research Committee of the Healthcare Financial Management Association (HFMA). At the time of the research being performed, discussed in chapters four, five and six, the author was a member of the committee. He became chair in 2020. In 2021, the author then became a Council member and Chair of the Public Policy and Reform Faculty Board of the Chartered Institute of Public Finance and Accountancy (CIPFA).

The role of these groups, and the broader NHS finance epistemic community, is relevant to this thesis, as is the overall approach of how to try to fuse the role of practice and research to try to influence and improve policy. An epistemic community is defined by Haas (2019) as:

> ...a network of professionals with recognised expertise and competence in a particular domain and an authoritative claim to policy-relevant knowledge within that domain or issue area. (Haas, 2019: 3)

HFMA is the association for finance practitioners in the UK NHS and has a stated aim of advising on health finance policy. CIPFA, as well as being the professional association which trains public sector accountants, also acts as the regulatory body for local government, and it also seeks to advise on public finance in all areas of public policy. Whilst there is considerable academic research in the NHS internal market field, outlined in Chapter 2, there is little practitioner research in health and care finance. This thesis contributes to filling this gap. Developing a greater understanding of the role of health finance professionals, which more clearly identifies their role in advising on the structures, and the funding approaches in place for the health and care system improvement is important. Potential improvements in approaches would help to ensure those structures and processes are delivering maximum value to the taxpayer and society. The role of professional groups and research is described in the work by Donald Schon (1983):

> According to the tradition of technical rationality, the professions mediate between science and society and translate scientific research into social progress. (Schon, 1983: 337)

In the context of health finance and policy, it is questionable how to direct this professional mediation is and how rapidly social progress is being made, noting the conclusions of Marmot et al (2020), and this will be described in this thesis. This could be because the finance practitioners do not see it as their role to advise on policy. They may see their role to implement policy, in a non-politicised way, akin to a view of the role of the wider civil service. However, as described in Chapter 5, the author has been involved nationally, via joint work between PwC and the HFMA, and elsewhere, which has tried to use practitioner views to directly inform policy and social progress.

There is a need for more practitioner research in health management and finance, and the role of academic research and policymakers can sometimes seem at odds as described by Greener et al (2014: 2):

> ...the dialogue between politicians, policymakers and academics engaged in research can be a series of miscommunications and misunderstandings. Academics appear to be engaged in spurious debates over arcane points that they spend their life writing about in unclear language, rarely saying what actually needs to be done, and policymakers trying to repeatedly reorganise public services based on little other than the belief that doing so will somehow make things better. There is now, for example, a great deal of evidence on the difficulties of achieving a successful structural healthcare reorganisation, but this doesn't seem to deter policymakers from engaging in yet another...healthcare reorganisation.

In summary, the current approach to the NHS internal market is being challenged, and the need for a change in public policy approach is considered by many long overdue. Therefore, the participants in the system need to help identify flaws with the current system, together with the consequence of those flaws and propose improved alternative approaches to organisations and how we organise and deliver services. Finance practitioners in health and care are in the middle of this policy landscape and this debate and therefore need to contribute more fully to it as reflexive practitioners. There is a need to try and bridge the gap between ill-evidenced practice and academic research.

The next chapter reviews the originating structure of the NHS and its foundations as a public service. It then reviews the development of the internal market in the English NHS. This provides a context to address the first two research questions around the funding approach and the impact of practitioner views on the market. It also then describes approaches to public policy implementation and the role of practitioners in public policy to provide a framework for answering the second and third research questions on how the attitudes of finance practitioners may be impacting policy implementation success and persistence and how finance practitioners should be participating in the development of policy.

CHAPTER 2

LITERATURE REVIEW: THE NHS, NEW PUBLIC MANAGEMENT, QUASI-MARKETS AND POLICY IMPLEMENTATION

This chapter describes the development of the NHS from its formation and then proceeds to describe the development of theory that supported an approach to state delivery through quasi-markets. In addition to describing the application of quasi-markets to the public sector, and specifically the English healthcare system, it also describes some analyses of the English NHS internal market, and some accounts of issues inherent in healthcare systems to further elaborate on the key conceptual problems impacting on this research including 1) measuring of system performance, 2) value and 3) wider determinants of disease, identified in Chapter 1. This chapter describes the development of the NHS market in England, as Scotland, Wales and Northern Ireland no longer have this market arrangement, and never implemented it in the same way as England did. The chapter also describes the process of public policy implementation to address the issues of how practitioners influence policy success and the overall policy environment itself.

2.1 The English NHS: History, Originating Structure and Development

The defining principle at the founding of the NHS was a widely held view of the need for, and the belief in the effectiveness of, state intervention in the health of the population. There was seen to be a role for the state in the delivery of healthcare improvement, which was prevalent in the politics of the time. The reasons for this are perhaps dependent upon that time, namely, there had been considerable success associated with collectivist state structures during the Second World War.

The development of the NHS was a large public policy undertaking and the scope and reach of its foundation should not be underestimated in terms of the changes it made. As Klein (2013: 1) noted, the foundation of the NHS in 1948 was the first health system in any Western society to offer free, comprehensive and national care. The birth of the NHS was a critical part of the Beveridge welfare reforms. Beveridge, a British economist, Liberal politician, and Director of the LSE, proposed finding ways of fighting the five "giants on the road of reconstruction" of Want, Disease, Ignorance, Squalor and Idleness, following the Second World War. Beveridge can be seen as a key architect of Britain's welfare system, of which the development of the NHS was a key component.

The formation of the NHS, to a large extent, defined the 1945 Labour Government, and much of the Keynesian-era social policy consensus up to the 1970s. The aims of the NHS Act in 1946 were to provide comprehensive access to healthcare services, based on need, not ability to pay, and were described by Glennerster (1995: 53) as follows:

- The service was to be run on a national basis and paid for out of general taxation.
- All citizens could register for free with a family doctor of their choice and receive free treatment for simple ailments and be referred to hospital for those conditions that the GP could not treat.
- GPs remained private professional people, increasingly often grouped in a common legal entity called a partnership.
- Attendance at hospital was free.
- Medicines prescribed by the GP could be picked up from the chemist for free. Eye tests and spectacles were free from the optician and visits to the dentist and fillings and other treatments were free too.

One of the struggles at the start of the NHS regarded the tension between the Labour Government and the medical profession which centred on the rights of doctors to continue to engage in private-sector treatment and care. This, along with mapping the new structure to the old, pre-existing structure, resulted in some compromise and was described by Brown and Payne (1990: 52):

> The administrative structure devised was a complicated tripartite one reflecting professional and administrative differences existing prior to 1946. The hospitals were 'nationalised' and they and the specialist services operating from within them were administered, under the Minister of Health, by a two-tier structure of regional hospital boards and hospital management committees. Local authorities gave up their hospitals but continued to provide environmental and community health services. The general practitioners continued to operate fairly independently but were under contract to local executive councils. The tripartite structure of the British health service was criticized almost from the inception of the NHS in 1946.

An ongoing debate since the NHS was first formed, therefore, has been about the best way to structure and manage the system of healthcare delivery to ensure the continuity of care between different parts of the service, and although steps have been taken to improve and develop the system, this debate on structure continues and is still highly relevant.

The defining nature of the NHS at its inception was to deal with absolute inequalities and unmet healthcare needs, particularly the poorest in society whose needs were not being met. However, in the context of the current debate about the NHS, an interesting feature is the view taken at the time on healthcare demand, as described by Ham (2009: 16):

> One of the assumptions that lay behind the NHS, and which had been made in the Beveridge Report, was that there was a fixed quantity of illness in the community, which the introduction of a health service, free at the point of consumption, would gradually reduce. It was therefore expected that expenditure would soon level off and even decline as people became healthier.

Given the ongoing debate about whether there is sufficient funding for the NHS, this view that the expenditure should soon level off and the decline has not been the experience of the service. A report for the House of Commons Library (see Figure 2.1) identified the growth in funding since 1948. Changes in technology and the ability of the NHS to intervene, along with the changing needs of the population can be seen as driving this increase in costs.

Figure 2.1: UK Expenditure on Health from Harker (2019)

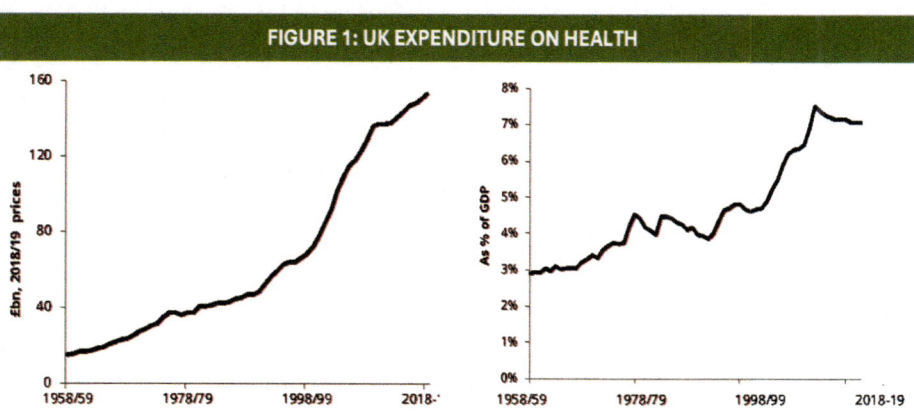

The costs of the NHS rose from around £11.4 billion in today's prices to over ten times that amount by 2018/19 at £152.9 billion (Harker, 2019: 3). A significant change to the NHS since its 1948 inception was attributable to the health reorganisation brought about by the Health Act in 1974. The period up to 1974 was one of relative stability, which started to be challenged in 1974 The relative stability in the NHS probably mirrored the post-war economic consensus around the role of the economy and the need for a supportive welfare state, that continued the Beveridge traditions.

The 1974 Act introduced Regional Health Authorities and District Health Authorities, to try and address the issues of the previous tripartite structure, as identified by Glennerster (1995), and it had two further ideas noted by Blakemore and Warwick-Booth (2013: 60):

> Reorganisation had three main aims. First, it was intended to unify health services by bringing under one authority all of the health services previously performed by regional Hospital Boards, Hospital Management Committees, boards of governors, executive councils and local health authorities. Unification was not, however, achieved in full because general practitioners remained independent contractors with the functions of executive councils being taken over by family practitioner committees. . . Second, reorganisation was intended to lead to better coordination between health authorities and local government services. . . A third stated aim of the reorganisation was to introduce better management.

In summary, the creation of the NHS is significant and was a key element of the Beveridge reforms of the welfare state and social policy. It was delivered at a time when there was a good deal of support for state intervention which continued for 30 years into the 1970s, and although there were refinements made to the approach to delivery and how the system was organised, there was broad political consensus on the approach.

The 1974 reorganisation sought to further "unify" provision, noting that the originating structure was the service was thought to be too fragmented. The NHS's first phase was defined by a collective belief in the role of the state to deliver improvements to the health and well-being of society. The 1974 reorganisation, however, was the first material change in the way in which the NHS was run and challenged the public policy orthodoxy of the times, and eventually led to the introduction of an internal market mechanism in the NHS. The underpinning of this internal market did not originate in the post-war political consensus. This author asserts that the introduction of this internal market can be traced to neo-liberal reactions to that post-war public policy. These reactions and their applications to the English NHS are described in the next section of this chapter.

2.2 New Public Management, Market Challenge and the NHS

Proponents of a market in health claim it would be less costly overall and deliver greater value. This approach was described by Allen and Sheaff (in Exworthy, Mannion and Powell, 2016: 212):

This doctrine suggests the construction of quasi-markets (Enthoven, 1985; Barlett and Le Grand 1993) in which the state, social insurer, or similar body purchases services on behalf of the consumer (Allen 2013) and in which plural providers of healthcare compete by stimulating innovation, improving healthcare quality and/or reducing costs.

Whether a true market's characteristics are exhibited in the English NHS quasi-market is contested. Markets tend to be the delivery mechanism of goods in the private sector and not a mechanism used in the public sector. As Lipsey (1989: 54) observed:

> The productive activity of a country is often subdivided in a different way to obtain the private and public sectors. The private sector refers to all the production that is in private hands, the public sector refers to all the production that is in public hands. The distinction between the two sectors depends on the legal distinction of ownership.

At a high level of characterising economies, those with all production in private hands are free market economies, and those where production is predominantly in public hands are considered state-controlled or socialist economies. All economies are, in reality, mixed economies with a combination of public and private ownership and provision. Markets tend to operate in the private sector and allocate resources optimally between suppliers and purchasers via managing volumes and prices. The application of markets into the public sector is a relatively new phenomenon.

New Public Management is underpinned by neo-liberal ideas. The most prominent early neo-liberal Friedrich von Hayek (1944) was keen to challenge the extended role of the state and revert back to a more liberal and libertarian society, which he believed would be more just and less oppressive.

> Even a good many economists with socialist views who have seriously studied the problems of central planning are now content to hope that a planned Society will have equal the efficiency of a competitive system; they advocate planning no longer because of its superior productivity but because it will enable us to secure a more just and equitable distribution of wealth. This is, indeed, the only argument for planning which can seriously be pressed. (Hayek (1944); 74)

Two key proponents of this neo-liberalism applied to administrative theory and public policy lie in the United States and two authors: William Niskanen and Gordon Tullock. Both authors describe the potential inefficiency of state provision of goods and services (those provided within public ownership) and are part of the Public Choice school of political economy. In Niskanen's case, the use of resources is claimed to be inefficient by the state provider and he describes the behaviour of bureaucracies. Niskanen makes claims that bureaus essentially begin to develop their own sets of objectives and then deliver services in accordance with their own bureaus' interests (for example increasing their size) as opposed to the interest of the populations and citizens they are designed to serve. Certainly, from the author's own perspective, it is an interesting challenge around the extent to which hospitals, and the wider NHS, serve their own organisational and bureaucratic needs, at the potential expense of the populations, they serve. Niskanen (1971: 227) noted:

> Most people, considering only their personal relationships with government, would prefer a government that is more efficient, more responsive, that generates larger total benefits, and for which the distribution of taxes and net benefits is more equitable. All of us who are concerned about the viability of our democratic political institutions and the integrity of our nation community would prefer a government with these attributes. The unavoidable conclusion…is that better government would be a smaller government.

Niskanen concludes that the potential behavioural and structural frailties of government bureaus give rise to the need to either (1) force the size of government down to a more optimal size; (2) create a competitive supply of public services; (3) allow national government to only supply core public services and allow local determination of the required level of public supply for non-core services; or (4) create a progressive tax system to achieve an equilibrium on the required supply of public services. The first three of these four "needs" were apparent in the challenge to the post-war consensus associated with the change in climate towards the NHS and the welfare state, around the time of the introduction of the NHS internal market, in the view of this author.

Tullock (2000) was equally distrustful of the role of Government. Public choice economists adopt a normative approach which characterises the actions of politicians, governments and bureaucracies as motivated by self-interest.

> Most public choice scholars do not think that the government is systematically engaged in maximising the public interest, but assume that the government officials are attempting to maximise their own private interests… My criticism of bureaucrats is, I should emphasise, not that they are bad people…It is the institutional situation in which they find themselves that frees them from the constraint of efficiently carrying out the tasks to which they have been assigned. (Tullock, 2000: 64)

The extent to which the neo-liberal and New Public Management approach to welfare delivery has systematically and coherently embedded itself in public policy related to the English NHS is open to question. Ferlie et al (1996) explored the complex nature of the implementation of New Public Management (NPM), noting the different strands of thinking within NPM including restructuring, quasi-markets, transformational change, the role of the Board and the interface with professionals and accountability. Despite this complexity, the notion of an internal market within the English NHS has prevailed and been sustained. And despite not privatising significant parts of delivery, and not introducing private health insurance or a wider role for a system of private medical facilities, these were discussed before the introduction of the internal market, and noted by Travis (2016: 1):

> The plan commissioned by Thatcher and her Chancellor suggests we have included proposals to charge for state schooling, introduced compulsory private health insurance and a system of private medical facilities that "would, of course, mean the end of the national health service".

The introduction of the internal market may therefore be seen as a political accommodation of neoliberal policy, without really changing more fundamentally moving towards private delivery, as described by Turner (2008). Perhaps the reason for the difficulty in implementing the internal market in health was the very same reason that it is now proving so difficult to dismantle.

> One general point is the effect of the bureaucratic and professional ownership within the state, which makes any attempt to reform policy a much longer process than was anticipated by neoliberal politicians. Specifically, in relation to health care plans for privatising the NHS would have been too costly and unpopular with the electorate. (Turner, 2008: 161)

Therefore, if there were plans to privatise the NHS, if that was the aim, these were seen as both costly and unpopular and were watered down. In addition, the difficulty in implementing a neo-liberal policy related to the NHS may also not just have been costs or popularity but could be seen in the length of time it takes to implement changes in public policy through a large bureaucratic structure. Today, ironically, it could be the slow pace at which the policy process itself can have an impact, given the size and the scale of the English NHS bureaucracy, that could now be preserving the internal market, that is leading to the policy's persistence.

Through the period 1989 to 2012, the NHS internal market had a coalition of Labour and Conservative support for it in England, or at least a lack of appetite to change the status quo of the internal market or an appreciation of the time it may take to implement a move away from it. Whether or not this represents the condition that Matland (1995) described as "policy clarity/low conflict" this author would question. Matland claims that policy implementation success requires the policy to be clear and there to be low levels of conflict to deliver it. This is discussed further in section 2.8. As Sabatier (1986: 42) observes:

> Major alterations in the policy core will normally be the product of changes external to the subsystem – particularly large-scale socio-economic perturbations or changes in the system-wide governing coalition. An example of the latter would be the change in Britain from Parliaments dominated by moderate socialists and conservatives to a system dominated by Mrs Thatcher's wing of the Conservative Party with a fundamentally different conception of the proper scope of Government activity.

Giddens (1986) attempted to try and reconcile these two competing views of the state and equity versus the market and economy. It could be argued that overall healthcare policy in this period has been defined by an apparent inability to marry and fuse these concepts. Giddens noted:

> ...no issue has polarised left and right more profoundly in recent years than the welfare state, extolled on the one side and excoriated on the other. What became "the welfare state" (a term not in widespread use until the 1960s and one William Beveridge, the architect of the British welfare state, thoroughly disliked) has in fact a chequered history. Its origins were far removed from the ideals of the left - indeed it was created partly to dispel the socialist menace...The welfare state as it exists today in Europe was produced in and by war, as with so many aspects of national citizenship. (Giddens, 1986: 111)

Hirschmann (1991) looks at the overall criticisms that have been made of the welfare state and wider state provision and categorises them. He puts these criticisms into three broad categories: the fact that progressive policy could cause jeopardy by undermining something else, the structures could cause a perverse impact by undermining the things they are trying to correct for, or the impacts of the approach could be futile, i.e., it is not possible to correct for the problem the progressive policy is trying to address.

> Surprisingly, the least effective argument against the welfare state has probably been the jeopardy thesis, which claims that the welfare state arrangements constitute a danger to individual liberties and

> to a properly functioning democratic society. In the more solidly established Western democracies, this argument has lacked credibility, except in some periods – such as the 1970s – when democratic institutions in several major countries appeared to be traversing a converging crisis. (Hirschmann, 1991: 138)

Irrespective of the political views of commentators, policymakers or other participants in the system, both managers and doctors, in either the public or private sector, need to be able to understand when their services are failing or are performing sub-optimally. Exworthy and Halford (1999) explore the relationship between the professions and NPM and describe the tension between the professional voice in public services and the NPM approach. The development of the internal market policy in health, coupled with the development of self-governing hospitals, could be seen to be responding to the concepts of 'exit' and 'voice' as two vehicles to better deliver through NPM. Hirschmann (1969) identifies these two ('exit' and 'voice') as the two major routes by which these failings – or suboptimal performances – may come to light. Either customers stop buying the products or leave the organisation as its goods or services are not good enough – 'exit'. Or the firm's customers or organisation's members express their dissatisfaction directly to management to try and elicit improvement or change – 'voice'. Both routes have continued to be applied in English NHS policy – 'exit' via the market mechanism, and 'choice' of GP, say; and 'voice' via the approach to Governing Bodies for Foundation Trusts or the role of Health and Wellbeing Boards or other forms of public and patient involvement currently embedded in the way in which the NHS is run.

In Tuohy (1999), the development and derivation of the healthcare public policy in the United States, Britain and Canada are contrasted and similarities are examined. Tuohy notes the different interest groups (patients, patient interest groups, the state itself, General Practitioners, hospital doctors, doctor professional associations, and even hospital managers) within each of the systems, and the nature of the way in which the public policy arena has developed over the course of the twentieth century, particularly contrasting the approaches to the development of the welfare state. From the development of the welfare state in the British system, Tuohy describes the development of the NHS and its "hierarchical corporatism" through to increased managerialism and the Griffiths Reforms, and then the relatively abrupt introduction of the internal market in the 1990s. The study stated that:

> . . . the most telling recognition of the extent to which the internal market reforms had been incorporated within the evolving logic of the British healthcare arena may have been the Labour Government's

decision to "go with the grain" in introducing its own set of policy proposals in 1997. The remarkable degree to which Labour moved from apocalyptic denunciation of the internal market reforms at the outset to acceptance of the basic features of the resulting model when it assumed power was not only a measure of ideological change in the Labour party with the rise of "New Labour". It was also a mark of the extent to which the internal market had become entrenched, as the key participants in the system accommodated to and shaped the reforms in the process of their implementation. (Tuohy, 1999: 202)

This account of the development of the approach to public policy development contextualises well the development of the internal market and its endurance. Tuohy notes public policy development as more incremental and based on a longer-range understanding of cultural and political phenomena, which accords with the author's view.

There may not, therefore, have been a clear and coherent policy framework for the internal market, but the implementation approach and methodology have been evolving with conflict around the policy due to the institutional dimensions Tuohy identifies. However, if there is a clear policy framework, it has a Public Choice theoretical underpinning and consequently has an impact on the approach to studying policy implementation. As Stoker (1995: 109) noted, British New Right think tanks such as the Institute for Economic Affairs and the Adam Smith Institute were keen to promote Public Choice inspired reform ideas associated with achieving 'optimal mechanism for allocating goods and making decisions is the market.' This was associated with a critique of the 'over-supply' of public services and insufficient responsiveness to individual consumers (Stoker, 1995). This critique was reflected in the endorsement of 'contracting out' by Oliver Letwin (1988: 77):

> The National Health Service has suffered extensive criticism as a result of its inadequate inspection of service standards when hospital cleaning and catering have been contracted out in some areas... Despite these problems, however, contracting out in Britain has genuinely been a success.

Whether or not the current policy landscape of the NHS can be traced back to New Public Management alone, itself in large part inspired by Public Choice ideas, is contested, however. Klein (2013) identified several different ways of describing the inception of the internal market through 'Working for Patients'. One description described the divergence away from the 1948 to 1989 medical establishment and government consensus, due to the then Prime Minister's view:

> Finally, bringing her exasperation to boiling point, she felt outraged when the Presidents of the Royal Colleges publicly denounced the government's policies. This represented, in her view, a repudiation of the implicit concordant between the state and the medical profession forged by the creation of the NHS, whereby the former accepted the autonomy of the medical profession in decisions about the use of resources while the latter accepted the right of the state to set the budgetary constraints within which it worked. (Klein, 2013: 141)

Whether or not the originating policy of the internal market represented a move towards privatisation of the actual clinical services or not is an interesting point and one which is very much contested. Certainly, at the outset of the policy, there were several options explored for changing the post-war settlement as further described by Klein (2013: 148):

> At the radical extreme were a number of proposals for privatising the finance of healthcare and giving the consumers the ability to choose between competing schemes by increasing the role of private insurance. The role of the state should be limited it was argued to ensure that everybody had the resources required to buy healthcare. Decisions about the appropriate level of spending on healthcare would largely be deemed depoliticised because diffused amongst consumers, the NHS budget would depend on its ability to attract customers in the face of competition from other providers. It was a model which had first been put forward 25 years previously by the Institute of Economic Affairs.

In the same way that the reasons for and the approach to the originating structure of the NHS are contested, there is a continued debate about what the internal market policy is now for or was introduced for. The author believes the quasi-market was an accommodation when the actual approach to the privatisation of the NHS did not seem politically acceptable, affordable, or practical. Pollock (2004) has offered a similar argument about the direction of travel of the internal market was intended to be privatisation. But, pertinent to this thesis, she also noted that the professionals inside the NHS who were managing the NHS were people with no background, training or experience in public health; instead, the system is populated at the top by:

> …arts graduates of all descriptions, ex-army officers, and, increasingly, people seeking a change from private enterprise (or surplus to its needs) - former chocolate and biscuits manufacturers, bank managers, Chief Executives of housing corporations. Many in this new management cadre are capable administrators but all of them - including those with some

substantial experience in the service - are now obliged to conform to an essentially business culture. (Pollock, 2004: 1)

Pollock, therefore, identified the new structure associated with the NHS as a key change in approach to both management and the participants in that management process and identifies it as being driven by ideology and a pathway to privatisation, rather than an evidenced, and necessarily required, change in policy course. According to Pollock, commodification and unbundling of the NHS's functions are important elements of the strategy for achieving the privatisation agenda. The internal market is hence a cornerstone of this process. Writers who assert that there is a privatisation agenda argue that the strategy outlined above has been followed by Conservative and Labour governments alike since the 1990s, although there are differences in how the internal market fits with a broader conception of how the NHS should operate. Leys and Player (2011), for example, noted that New Labour imagined that a 'managed market' could emerge with the state playing an important role in shaping the internal market system, while the Conservative-led coalition government wanted to advance a more assertive market with a much-reduced role for the Secretary of State, reflected in the 2012 Act. While there were differences of interpretation and emphasis, the role of the internal market was not seriously questioned.

While it is important to understand the changing nature of national policy agendas, as will be discussed below, this thesis asserts the importance of also understanding the 'worldviews' of the participants in the NHS internal market. If one believes that those individuals delivering state services are motivated by notions of public service and accountability, then state provision can be effective, and the need for a competitive market diminishes. If there is a need to correct for the private interest of bureaucrats, the need for a market is intensified. Whether there is an internal market in health to achieve a privatised system, or an internal market within the public sector, or whether there is an internal market in name alone, is subject to significant debate around the principles, the rationale, and the reality of the policy.

2.3 The Development of the Market in the English NHS

The Griffiths Report (1983) sought to make the NHS more "business-like" via the introduction of general managers at all levels of the NHS. Prior to this point, Griffiths, a former deputy Chairman and Managing Director of Sainsbury's, concluded there had been poor general management skills within the NHS, which he sought to address, with the backing of the Secretary of State for Health.

> Absence of this general management support means that there is no driving force seeking and accepting direct and personal responsibility for developing management plans, securing implementation and monitoring actual achievement. It means that the process of devolution of responsibility to the Units, is far too slow. (Griffiths 1983: 1)

Beyond this development of greater managerialism within NHS structures, the next move saw revisions to the structures themselves via the development of a purchaser/provider split in that management, which could potentially assist doctors and management to run their services mindful of the motivations and impacts of potential 'exit'. In addition, the "Working for Patients" (1989) White Paper had seven overall aims, of which the first three are listed, below:

> First: to make the Health Service more responsive to the needs of patients, as much power and responsibility as possible will be delegated to local level.
>
> Second: to stimulate a better service to the patient, hospitals will be able to apply for a new self-governing status as NHS Hospital Trusts.
>
> Third: to enable hospitals which best meet the needs and wishes of patients to get the money to do so, the money required to treat patients will be able to cross administrative boundaries. (DoH, 1989: 4)

Prior to the 1989 White Paper, the English NHS had been managed through integrated health bodies called District Health Authorities (DHAs) which controlled and managed both hospitals and other parts of the NHS including the funding to GPs, dentists and direct control and management of other parts of the NHS system. Many commentators note the impact of "Working for Patients" on the NHS system. For example, Ham (2009: 41) notes that the move from DHAs to 'a contract system in which responsibility for purchasing and provision was separated. This was achieved by the creation of entirely new organisations – self-governing NHS trusts – to manage services thereby enabling DHAs to focus on purchasing healthcare for the populations they served.'

This signalled a key shift in the development of public policy with a belief that the new 'market' system (although 'Working for Patients' avoided using the word 'market' word at all), would, to some extent, challenge the producer interests of hospitals by creating a payment formula linked to work completed, not historic budgets, and drive further improved performance, by the choice of hospital, by patients and their General Practitioners:

> The Government believes that these new funding arrangements will bring down waiting times for hospital treatment. They will move money to where the work is best done and will make maximum waiting times an important feature of contracts and management budgets. (DoH 1989: 37)

The 'Working for Patients' White paper contained other policy changes that still reside in the current English NHS policy landscape:

- Further development of the management of the system building from the Griffith's Report.
- Self-governing hospitals continue today via self-governing Foundation Trusts.
- The development of a fee-for-service model of funding for hospitals, for work completed as opposed to funding based on historic budgets, which continued up to the pandemic.
- Reforms to the payment of hospital consultants to try and ensure there is greater accountability for their actions.
- Patient choice is built from the patient's relationship with their GP.
- The funding mechanism for GPs and Family Health Services is based on a capitation formula.
- Improving governance and accountability for Regional Health Authority structures.
- Permissions is given for working more closely with the private sector in the delivery of services.

'Working for Patients' is therefore the antecedent of many of the current quasi-market structures in health, which are maintained in the English NHS up to the present day despite the 2022 Act. Although there have been further developments, they have largely tweaked the 'Working for Patients' formula, as opposed to having overhauled it. It was not until the 2012 Health Act, which removed the Strategic Health Authorities that anything had materially changed in the overall approach to the management structures of the English NHS. Importantly, from 1989 to 2022, each incarnation of the internal market has relied upon a belief in the role of competition between secondary care providers and that this will lead to greater system efficiency.

The second major overhaul of the internal market happened around 2005 and was signalled by 'Creating a Patient-led NHS'. The policy document looked for choice for patients (in line with other public sector reforms), with integrated networks of care for certain types of care, urging Primary Care Trusts (PCTs) to promote choice for acute care, developing the Foundation Trust approach and seeking the further development of PCTs.

The policy document particularly sought to improve services through the idea of patient choice. There were then seen to be three further levers driving change in the NHS system. First, improvement to a system of payment for services via transactional reform. Second, supply-side reforms were seen as necessary with a more plural market for provision including Foundation Trust, non-Foundation Trust and nationally procured Independent Sector Treatment Centres, which the policy particularly heralded. Third, was the idea of system management reforms which sought to improve the regulatory environment for health with the development of Monitor as the economic regulator, and the Healthcare Commission as the quality regulator. The reforms were articulated with the use of the diagram Figure 2.2.

Figure 2.2 - Health Reform in 2005 – Diagrammatic Representation

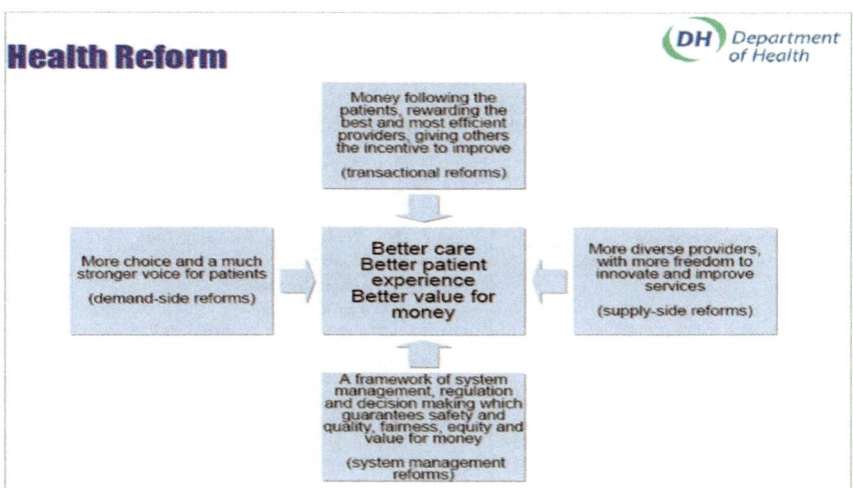

These further reforms built more of an infrastructure to deliver the 'Working for Patients' model including a continued focus on managerialism, self-governing hospitals, fee for hospital service, payment reforms for hospital consultants, patient choice, capitation funding for primary care, improved governance and accountability and the use of the private sector. During the author's NHS career to date, these are all concepts which have been prevalent in the NHS management and finance and have, from a finance and wider managerial practitioner perspective, remained largely uncontested, since 1989. The epistemic groups within the NHS finance community of either HFMA or CIPFA have not overtly called for a policy change and have, in the author's opinion, tended to lag the emerging and then prevailing policy of the time.

It was the 2005 reforms that saw many of the currently existing statutory structures put in place, including the Care Quality Commission (CQC), and the further Quasi-Autonomous Non-Government Organisation (QuANGO) named Monitor, as the quality and provider regulators for health services. The mixed economy of providers included the more independent Foundation Trusts then regulated by Monitor and non-FTs under the control of ten Strategic Health Authorities (SHAs), with Primary Care Trusts (PCTs) the latest name (then) for the local commissioning bodies.

Research by Ham and others has described the 'Working for Patients' quasi-market, as Market 1 (1991-1997). The quasi-market associated with 'Creating a Patient-Led NHS' is described as Market 2 (2002-2010). The intervening periods have still seen a market in operation. Although the public policy emphasis on markets has waxed and waned over the three decades since 1989, three key components have remained unchanged: 1) delegation of power (the extent of this has been challenged by some commentators), 2) self-governing hospitals, and 3) money following the patient.

Table 2.1 - Differences between the 1991 and 2002 market reforms (Ham, 2009: 9)

NHS market, 1991-1997 – 'Market 1' - Patient choice restricted to fundholding GPs	NHS market, 2002 – 2010 – 'Market 2' - Patient Choice of Elective Provider
Health Authority Purchasing - Contracts not subject to contract law	**Primary Care Trust (PCT) commissioning** - Contracts legally binding
Fundholding - Voluntary - Fundholders able to retain surpluses	**Practice-based commissioning** - Universal, at least for PCTs - Intention that any surpluses be shared with PCTs
NHS Trusts - Some price competition - Unable to retain surpluses - In practice, access to new sources of capital restricted and not free to borrow commercially	**Foundation trusts** - Paid increasingly using fixed prices under Payments by Results - Surpluses can be retained to reinvest - Commercial borrowing within limits
Evaluation - No independent studies until late in the reform process	**Evaluation** - Programme of independent evaluation studies commission by Department of Health

Table 2.1 notes the key differences between the two phases of quasi-market development. 'Market 2' made the system more legally enshrined via the enforceability of legal contracts. Although, 'Market 2' saw legal contracts enforceable in law, there has never been a legal challenge to an intra-NHS contract, as practitioners largely believe, it would be a waste of taxpayers' money and bring the NHS into disrepute. Practitioners tended to believe that if they followed this route, it may equate to just moving money within parts of the same DHSC budget and spending its resources on unnecessary legal fees.

The policy developed through 'Creating a Patient-led NHS', with Market 2 (2002-2010) was reviewed by Mays, Dixon and Jones (2011) for the Kings'

Fund. Potentially to its credit, "Creating a patient-led NHS" did call for an evaluation of the internal market approach. The review noted:

> Although the effects of the Labour government's market reforms (2002 – 2010) . . . are not dramatic, there is evidence to suggest that they were beginning to have some positive impact. However, almost nothing is known about the costs of competition, or its relative effect compared to other approaches such as targets and performance management. The issue, then, for policymakers is whether the costs both financial and political, are worth the effort, if these reforms achieve limited change. (Mays et al, 2011; 160)

Even though the prevailing public policy orthodoxy for the English NHS has been an internal market, the evidence for its derivation and efficacy in policy terms is not conclusive. The positive impact described by Mays et al was thought to include a choice of provider for elective services but then went on to note:

> If the priority is now to make the health system more responsive to the needs of those with ongoing physical and mental health needs, then competition may need to be complemented by other approaches (e.g., various forms of so-called integrated care.) (Mays et al, 2011: 160)

Since 1989 a good deal of modification to the policy has occurred, seeing a widening of choice, legally binding contracts, attempts at increasing doctor involvement with commissioning or purchasing, and even more independence for hospitals, via the Foundation Trust movement. The original creation, and continuing maintenance, of this structure was not an easy task. This point was noted by Klein (2013):

> The government had provided a bold, outline sketch…But long after the official launch in April 1991, the managerial engineers were still working hard plugging the leaks and adapting the design even when the ship was lurching through heavy seas. Of necessity the NHS became a learning system, inventing itself as it went along. (Klein, 2013: 161).

The assertions by many neo-liberals that a market-like approach would spontaneously emerge and hence could reduce the direct role of the government in managing health was shown to be flawed. Even the logic of devolving decision-making in the NHS to engage in blame-shifting for the allocation and use of resources was shown to be problematic and resulted in more, not less, intervention from the centre. (Klein, 2013: 169).

Klein (2013) notes that the implementation of the NPM in English healthcare was difficult and contested. Walsh et al (1997) noted the evolving approach to markets and contracting in UK public services. Although this work did not claim to be a systematic evaluation of the whole policy area, they support the view that some of the approaches to NPM contracting go with the grain of human behaviour and some do not, some are consistent with democratic decision making and others not, and some may lead to better outcomes but they overall question whether market-driven approaches will always (or usually) meet their objectives.

2.4 2012 Health Act and Quasi – 'Market 3'

Although never referred to in either the Conservative or Liberal Democrat manifestos in advance of the Coalition Government, a further embedding of the market, in the NHS, was proposed by the Coalition Government. The further development and solidification of the internal market was a central pillar of the 2012 Health Act. Although the Act was subject to a "pause" in the legislative process, due to the House of Lords and wider opposition to it, and watered down the original intent, 'Market 3', specifically, included (as summarised from Lamb, 2012): (a) a new role for Monitor, as the economic regulator of healthcare, (b) removal of Foundation Trusts Private Patient cap, (c) more freedom for Foundation Trusts on their constitutions, (d) new statutory fiduciary duties for Directors of Foundation Trusts similar to those in the 2006 Companies Act, (e) changes to Foundation Trust governance whereby the Council of Governors are to hold the non-executive directors to account, (f) Foundation Trust Board of Directors to meet in public unless there are "special reasons", (g) changes to the regulation of mergers and acquisitions within healthcare, (h) the development of a new failure regime for Foundation Trusts, and (i) changes in the transparency of financial assistance given to Foundation and other Trusts in the system.

The 2012 Health Act, therefore, built more market phraseology and mechanisms into the 1989 system and could be seen as a logical extension of those changes. There was a move towards more formal economic regulation between the revised role of Monitor and the links to the Competition and Markets Authority to ensure effective market-based delivery. More freedoms and equivalent private sector duties for the Boards of Foundation Trust hospitals were introduced. A more "private sector" model for mergers and acquisition, a failure regime for healthcare providers, and a growing transparency around the funding hospitals were increasingly receiving from the DoH, beyond the Payment by Results fee-for-service system. Increasingly, during this period, several NHS Provider organisations were in receipt of special payments from the DoH to keep paying their bills and delivering their services, beyond those which they were formally eligible for under the PbR system. Also, the 2012 Act saw the removal of the ten strategic health authorities, to remove some management costs from the system. This was the first time since the inception of the NHS that no sub-national coordinating body for health services had existed, a change signalling, perhaps, further faith in the market approach.

The 2012 Health Act was a particularly fraught piece of legislation. Although the legislation may be seen as a continuance of that which had gone before, the opposition to the Bill was considerable. Increasingly voices were being heard about the potential lack of effectiveness of commissioning structures and whether they worked. This was increasingly apparent with the professional network of which the author is part, but also more generally. For example, a cross-party House of Commons Select Committee Report (2010: 3) noted that commissioning had not lived up to its promise in the two decades since 'Working for Patients':

> Whatever the benefits of the purchaser/provider split, it has led to an increase in transaction costs, notably management and administration costs. Research commissioned by the DoH but not published by it estimated these to be as high as 14% of total NHS costs. We are dismayed that the Department has not provided us with clear and consistent data on transaction costs; the suspicion must remain that the DH does not want the full story to be revealed. We were appalled that four of the most senior civil servants in the Department of Health were unable to give us accurate figures for staffing levels and costs dedicated to commissioning and billing in PCTs and provider NHS trusts.

Timmins (2012: 2) has described the somewhat unusual passage of the 2012 Act to the statute book, which was extraordinary, compared to the normal legislative assent process.

> So great was the resistance – not least from the grassroots of the coalition – that the Government was forced into an unprecedented 'pause' over its legislation. The pause however failed to silence the critics. There were times when it looked like the Bill would be lost. In fact, it got through.

There were many other changes associated with the Health Act 2012 impacting the further development of the English NHS Market, particularly in terms of changes around commissioning. There were changing structures proposed for commissioning with the dissolution of the Primary Care Trusts, to be replaced with Clinical Commissioning Groups (CCGs). This was a large-scale institutional change in health organisations, which was not heralded by either the Conservative or Liberal Democrat manifestoes. One of the results of the extended pause on the legislation, following its passage through Parliament, was a parallel duty on the participants in the internal market system to cooperate as well as compete. What a "cooperative market" is, in the context of New Public Management, as an economic or market theory is open to question. This addendum to the original Bill's intention can be seen as an accommodation and dilution of the intended policy, due to the "pause". The policy environment has therefore moved on again, but the market mechanisms and the split between commissioning and provision have remained.

The precise changes associated with the Bill, described above, were many; and there has been no primary legislation on health reorganisation between the 2012 Act and the 2022 Act. It is interesting now to reflect on the extent to which the opposition to the 2012 Act which generated the 'pause' was due to the political uproar over the fact that no primary legislation was planned by either coalition manifestos, or due to the growing impatience with the market structures in health, which this Act was a further incarnation of. Even though this was a continuation of the market policy, the 2012 Act can still be seen as a significant change to how the services were run.

> Their work was to be overseen by a new national commissioning board. The entire existing superstructure of the NHS (the 10 regional health authorities and 152 primary care trusts) was to be abolished. (Timmins, 2012: 15)

In addition to these high-level changes, a new economic regulator was planned to oversee extended choice and competition. An "any willing provider" model was to be introduced to enable easier change in the supply of care. Also, the existing public health body, the Health Protection Agency was to be absorbed into the DoH, and a large amount of the public health budget was transferred to local authorities. Health and Well-being Boards were to be created in local government to try to join up the commissioning of NHS services, social care and prevention. And a new patient voice organisation, Healthwatch, was to be created.

The 2012 Act was a large shift in power and accountability, with GPs required to be positioned in the driving seat of commissioning, while whole tiers of existing management of the NHS were to be abolished. Further, one of the phenomena introduced in the 2012 Act was a formalised "failure regime" for English NHS provider organisations. Over the period of Market 2, there had become a series of emerging financial problems in individual providers which needed some sort of answer to the following question: "What happens to NHS provider organisations who can no longer operate within the level of funding afforded to them by the English NHS provider funding formula?". The nature of that funding formula is described in Chapter 3, but the outcome of the use of the failure regime is of interest in terms of how embedded a market approach had or had not become.

The Failure Regime in England has been used twice since the 2012 Health Act was introduced. Along similar lines to that which the insolvency regime is used in the private sector a special administrator is appointed to wind up the failing organisation. The first instance was used for Mid Staffordshire Hospital in Staffordshire, due to several care failings, which sent a large shockwave across the NHS system. The second was in the case of South London Healthcare, which had a Trust which had poor financial health caused not least by Greenwich Hospital being home to an early PFI for its new hospital. The two Trust Special Administration Reports (2012 and 2013) proposed relatively modest changes to clinical services and a need for increased funding for the two sites. Additional funding is not the likely outcome of receivership in the private sector and perhaps is highly illustrative of the weakness of the English NHS internal market to deliver allocative efficiency through competition, and consequent market exit through failure. It is important to note that pre-pandemic the growing number of provider hospital organisations' deficits did not result in further uses of the failure regime and that practitioners within health finance noted how unaffordable the continued use of the failure regime could be.

The 2012 Act, therefore, saw a continuation of market policy, at the point at which there was the most coherent set of voices, via the Health Select Committee and other opponents to the Bill, to the market itself. Elements of the epistemic communities in NHS finance that this thesis explores were also beginning to voice concerns. There was therefore further thinking within professional practice which questioned the market's efficacy and asked whether a different delivery structure was needed to replace the purchaser/provider split.

2.5 Assessing the Internal Market and Current Management Arrangements and Views on their Replacement.

The problem with assessing the impact of the NHS internal market is that the internal market strand of public policy does not operate in isolation in the English NHS. Over the period of Market 1, Market 2, and Market 3, strands of policy related to the delivery of targets and goals, set by the DoH coexist. The extent to which the system is therefore changing due to the market structures, the targets set, or other factors is therefore hard to discern and separate.

Allen (2012) builds on the work of Tuohy (1999), by drawing out Tuohy's analytical concepts of structural dimensions in health, state, private finance and professions. The state tends to operate through a structure of "hierarchy and control", whereas private finance operates through a "market"; and the professions in healthcare, particularly identifying the medical profession, (although the author would identify wider professional groupings in health in this category, including NHS managers and finance practitioners), tend to operate through a system which is described as "collegiality". Allen then further noted that the institutional dimensions tend to drive how the structural dimensions operate. In this way, it could be asserted that the English NHS is operating through three different structural and institutional dimensions (Allen, 2012: 289):

1. The structure of any particular healthcare system is context and path-dependent, bound by decisions in the distant past (See Pierson, 2000).

2. The importance of interrelationships between different interest groups (such as the state, private finance and the medical profession) and the different institutions (such as the market, hierarchy and professional networks) for understanding the dynamics of policy-making and delivery in the healthcare system.

3. The enduring role of the state and its hierarchies for the operation of the NHS in England.

The difficulty in assessing the NHS internal market therefore can be described as multi-faceted. Given the policy is complex, it is hard for the researcher to define the policy in play, and then assess the policy implementation (given the number of actors in the system). Furthermore, how does the researcher describe the impact of the system itself on the delivery of policy (given its complex nature and multiple structures, interest groups and institutions)?

The extent to which the rhetoric of the market was prevalent or whether a 'real' market has been and is in operation is at issue also, but certainly, the language of a market system has remained reasonably intact during the period from 1989 to the current date. Paton (1998) discusses the 'what is the reality of the internal market' line of inquiry. He asserts that the reforms are probably not rationally designed to meet long-term public policy objectives, but they may be part of an ongoing struggle in the public policy of the UK, around the use of internal markets in the NHS, and potential privatisation.

> To make this point sharply: were the reforms merely the most recent in an increasingly long line of administrative reorganisations within

the National Health Service or are they an enabling catalyst for the abandonment of consensus around the provision of a universal, comprehensive and egalitarian public health service? (Paton, 1998: 7)

The study of the English NHS almost, therefore, cleaves into i) a slightly more questioning narrative account of the phenomena involved, versus ii) an attempt to try and review the effectiveness of the approach adopted, assuming an internal market as a relatively coherent policy objective has been created. Difficulties with appraising the evidence, include (a) lack of a programme of evaluation of changes made, (b) lack of clarity around what the reforms were meant to deliver, (c) the confounding effects of other factors, and (d) the difficulty of selecting a methodology to appraise success. Le Grand et al (1998: 137) noted:

> But all of this begs the fundamental question of whether there should be competition at all. Here our review of the evidence offers little help. Because, in practice, competition was patchy, we do not know, on balance, whether its impact was detrimental or beneficial – or what the consequences would have been if it had been extended.

In the English NHS, we continue with a purchaser/provider split and a good deal of contention around the extent to which there is really an internal market in operation. The 'Market 3' structural architecture of the NHS was supported by a complex financial structure. In the wake of the 2012 Health Act, there were 211 CCGs, and NHS England was directly responsible for commissioning some elements of healthcare. There was then a series of regulators with an oversight role to assure quality or sound financial provider behaviour. There were around 250 NHS provider organisations delivering care, ignoring the continuing independent contractor status of most GPs. In addition, there was a body, Health Education England, responsible for training doctors and nurses. Also, there was Public Health England which worked with local government on the public health and well-being agenda. Local government had these local public health responsibilities transferred to it in the 2012 Act. The 2022 Act has changed the structures further in England, mainly incorporating Public Health England, Health Education England and NHSI, into NHSE; and replaced the former CCGs with 42 ICBs. Figure 2.3, from the British Medical Journal, also noted the differences between the English versus Scottish, Welsh and Northern Ireland systems.

Figure 2.3 - Into the labyrinth: BMJ (2017) UK health and social care funding

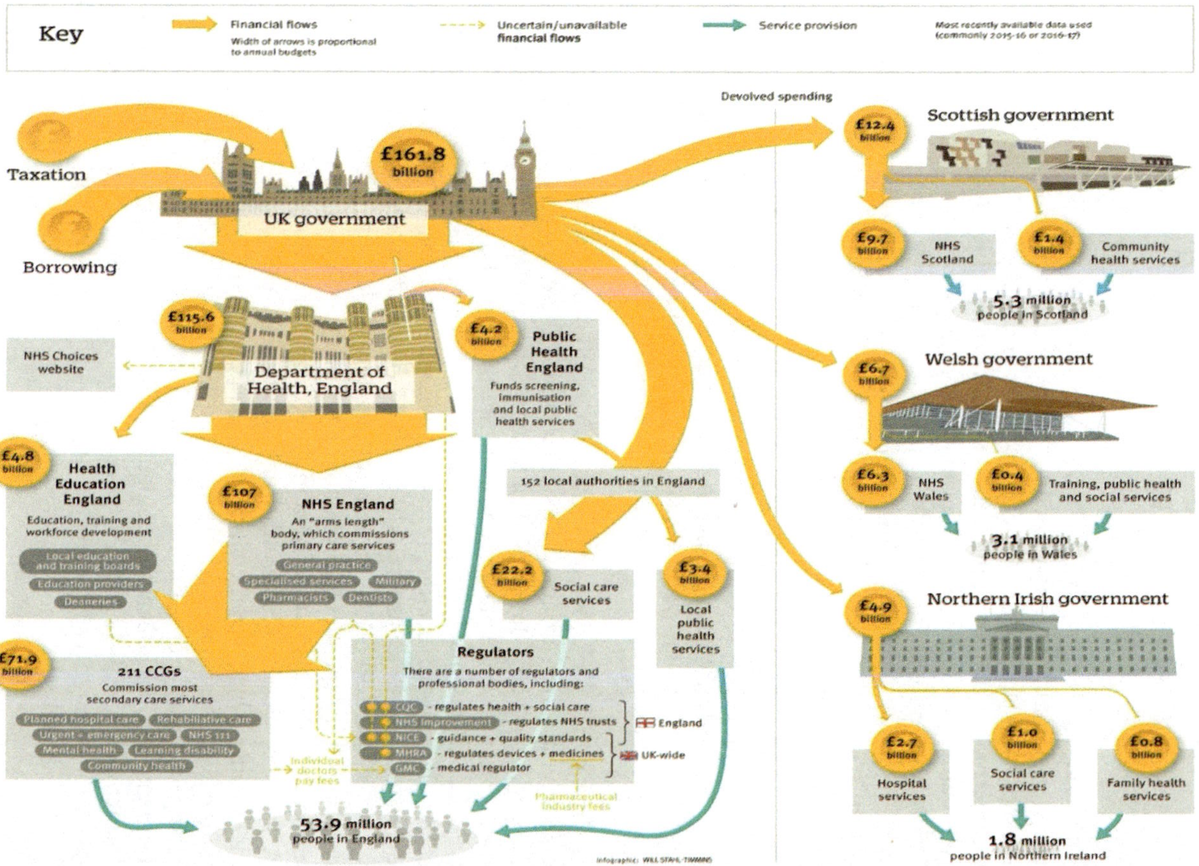

If we take just a view of the English system prior to 2022 for illustration, Figure 2.4 shows the connections between the Parliament, Government, Secretary of State, then NHS England, NHS Improvement, and the Care Quality Commission, before getting to the contractual relationships between purchasers and providers. This chart shows the partners to the Sustainability and Transformation Plans (STPs) – Local Authorities, Clinical Commissioning Groups and NHS providers. These STPs (latterly Partnerships) were a previous attempt to try and better link together the organisations in a particular geography that deliver and develop the care services. These non-statutory structures were developed following the 2012 Health and Social Care Act but were not part of it. As Alderwick et al (2016: 4) commented:

> Sustainability and transformation plans (STPs) are plans for the future of health and care services in England. NHS organisations in different parts of the country have been asked to collaborate to respond to the challenges facing local services. This marks a decisive shift from the focus on competition as a means of improving health service performance in the Health and Social Care Act 2012.

Figure 2.4 – HFMA - The "current" England 2018 NHS structure and organisations

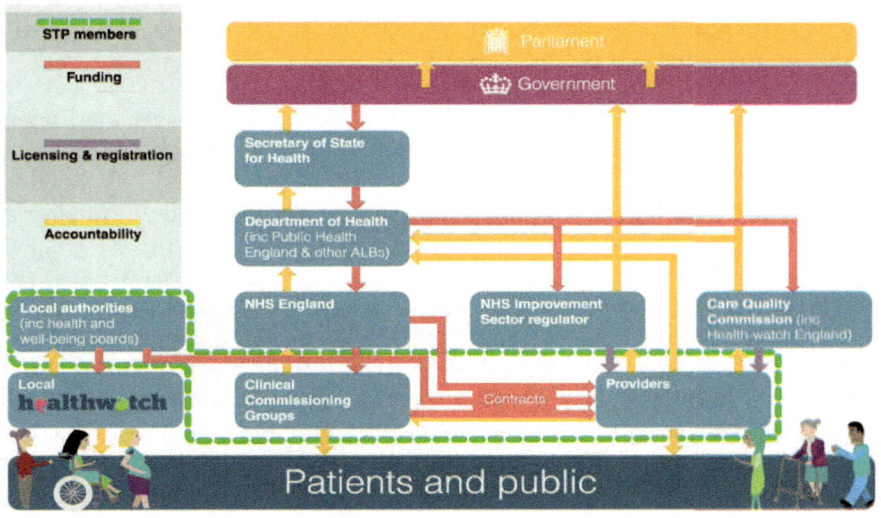

Whilst trying to assess the performance of the market structure, it is therefore important to note that there is now a broad coalition which is talking about the need to change these structures. But there is considerable resistance from various interests against this, including managers. Mintzberg (2017) notes that there are several myths which have crept into health service management which need to be challenged.

> Myths abound…in what is called the system of healthcare, not least that it is a system that is about the care of health. Combine these … myths and you get what we have: a non-system that is being managed out of control. (Mintzberg, 2017: 9)

Mintzberg summarises these myths into nine:

#1 that we have a system of healthcare.

#2 that this system is failing.

#3 that it can be fixed with heroic leadership.

#4 with more administrative engineering.

#5 with more categorising and commodifying to facilitate more calculating.

#6 with an increased level of competition.

#7 by managing it more like a business.

#8 that healthcare is rightly left to the private sector for the sake of efficiency and choice.

#9 or rightly controlled by the public sector for the sake of equality and economy.

Mintzberg essentially debunks much of the public policy narrative which has surrounded the English NHS since 1989. He notes that the system of health has become increasingly successful, if costly, due to drug and wider treatment success, and that the narrative of failure is of interest in the context of the success of demonstrably falling mortality rates in many countries. Mintzberg (2017: 75) argues critically both against the use of competition and against more solutions which surround managing health more like a business.

> …in the United States, where competition is probably the greatest, and so too are these beliefs, competition has more likely done more harm than good in healthcare; and second, that healthcare everywhere, already has too much competition, but of a kind less recognised – it requires a good deal more cooperation.

The American system spends significantly more of its GDP on healthcare, and it also has worse outcomes in many instances, than several other comparative countries, as previously noted in the Commonwealth Fund comparative studies. It also, as a society has an attitude towards business which could be regarded as more deferential, as Mintzberg (2017: 87) noted:

> When it comes to managing everything, this is a prevailing myth in our societies, especially in the U.S., that business has it right while most other institutions, especially government, have it wrong. Therefore, all must ape business, if not actually become businesses. . . Across government services, this agenda has been promoted as the "New Public Management" … As a consequence, much of the public sector now ambles about like an amnesiac pretending to be business.

There are many factors at play when addressing whether the internal market in the English NHS continues to be relevant and/or successful. The extent to which we are adhering to some mythology about business or competitive structures is important. Following the 2012 Act, which gave the NHS a greater degree of business and competitive mechanisms and removed a coordinating tier of the English NHS system, there was a move to even more competitive structures and rhetoric.

Despite the author's long-held beliefs on the efficacy and lack of requirement for an internal market in health, there continue to be proponents of the 'competition will generate efficiency' view, particularly from the US. Porter and Tiesberg (2006: 324) are such proponents:

> Health care policy is highly controversial, with strong advocates for widely differing models: a government-controlled national health care system, a single-payer system, a consolidation into integrated health systems combining a health plan with a captive full-line provider network, or a consumer-driven system in which the consumers bear personal responsibility for cost . . . A government-run system can allow for universal coverage and tight cost control but will eliminate competition altogether and worsen the problems with the value of care that plague the current system. Government-run health systems in other parts of the world are encountering increasing problems with quality, costs and rationing.

The need for competition in health is put centre stage here. One could easily claim that the need or not for competition in health is a subjective judgement, based on a fundamental belief in the relative efficacy or not of the state to be able to deliver certain goods or services, in a more advantageous way than a market mechanism. Porter and Teisberg (2006: 382) continue:

> When Providers succeed in delivering superb care more efficiently, patients, health plans and employers also succeed. When health plans help patients and referring clinicians make better-informed choices, seek out superior care, and assist in the coordination of care, excellent providers also benefit. Competing on value also goes beyond economic success. When physicians and health professionals compete to achieve the best outcomes for patients, they pursue the aims that led them into the profession in the first place. No longer are economic realities and personal values in conflict.

Whether competition in health is good or bad takes some teasing out before deciding, but it must be based on the circumstances and context in which the healthcare system operates. Such attempts have been made. A relatively early international comparative study of markets in healthcare was attempted by Ranade et al (1998: 212) and concluded:

> Whether the market will go on rising in healthcare, or whether it is yesterday's story, is still open to question, depending on how healthcare fits into the political economy and social culture of each country. The reasons lie in the twin face of healthcare: as a core function of the welfare state and an industry of massive proportions...The reshaping of the healthcare state is inextricably caught up in the wider welfare and industrial restructuring precipitated by the emerging dynamics of global capitalism and the struggles for national competitiveness. The balance between market forces and welfare values in healthcare will depend on how these struggles are resolved.

There is also contention in the English NHS market about the use of both the language and ethnography associated with the NHS reform process. "Simple terms" such as governance, choice, freedom and accountability are observed to have multiple and ambiguous meanings. Morrell (2006: 379) notes:

> The policy literature on NHS reform glosses over the inherent complexities in understanding, accountability and governance in healthcare. A number of normative elements are evident in the literature, and they can be located in a narrative which references three themes: the self-evident need to change, the promise of liberation, and the signalling of moral duties and responsibility.

Cooper et al (2012) studied whether or not competition increased hospital efficiency in the English NHS and created a reaction on the actual meaning of the work, and the extent to which the work was without bias. They observed:

> First, our findings demonstrate that hospital competition can lead to improvements in public providers' productivity based on our observed reductions in hospitals' pre-surgical Length of Stay... While we did find that competition improved providers' productivity, we also found that there is a real risk that hospital competition between general hospitals and specialty surgical centres can lead to risk segmentation, with large incumbent hospitals at risk of inheriting a riskier patient case mix who are more costly to treat. (Cooper, Gibbons, Jones and McGuire, 2012: 24)

Pollock et al (2012) noted in response to the paper and the ongoing media debate that followed it during the period around the "pause" on the Health and Social Care Bill and a more general debate on the NHS market:

> Le Grand and Cooper call themselves "empiricists" and all those that disagree with them "intuitivists". Unlike scientists, however, they have made no "real life" observations themselves from which they have generated their theories... Bad science makes bad policy and bad policy leads to careless talk. Careless talk will cost lives especially when it is used in support of the HSC Bill. (Pollock, MacFarlane and Greener, 2012: 3)

Given this struggle, it is relatively rare to find academic literature which makes specific recommendations on how to change healthcare systems or the English NHS. Paton (2016) evaluates the health reforms of the last thirty years and notes the differential implementation of the reforms across the UK. He proposed a:

> ...more economic approach to management and governance, with a better chance of achieving care which is planned to suit the patient's needs in the most appropriate location at different stages of illness or need. One organisation which holds the responsibility for care is more likely to design 'care pathways' with the correct incentives to staff across the pathway. That is a lesson from the USA, where the most cost-effective Healthcare Maintenance Organisations have done this. (Paton, 2016: 202)

Paton's recommendations are abridged in Table 2.2 and there are several interesting dimensions to his proposals from the author's perspective. They correlate to some of the proposals made regarding practitioner views described further in Chapter 5. The area which is perhaps slightly less radical concerns

GPs, from this author's perspective. There is a growing trend for hospital Trusts and others to run GP practices. GPs provide services as well as have a commissioning role from 2002 to 2022. Without a clearer management and clinical understanding of the care boundaries between community services, mental health services and the role of primary care, the proposals may not quite go far enough. Also, the proposal is relatively silent on the interrelationships between health and local government. Without a clearer relationship between the health bodies and local government - which the STPs have sought to address (and how the ICBs are seeking to further address), there are these continued fractures in the health and care system. Paton's proposals relate to streamlining many elements of the current England NHS structure are to be welcomed, though. It could be noted that the 2022 Act delivered the Paton "Blueprint" apart from the proposed further Provider side reforms.

Table 2.2 - A Blueprint to map the current 'market' to a tidied up English NHS (Paton (2016); 197)

Current	Proposal
Commissioning CCG's	Abolished
Community NHS Trusts	Absorbed geographically into hospital Trusts Absorbed geographically into hospital Trusts
Hospital Trusts	Become geography based integrated providers
Mental Health Trusts	Become a division in the integrated provider
GPs	Allowed to refer to any integrated provider
Regional Officers (four - NHSE and NHSI)	Regional Health Authorities (RHAs) - ten which plan services regionally
CQC, Monitor/TDA (now NHSI)	Merged into one authority quality and governance could be called NHS Governance
NHSE	Now responsible for the whole of the NHS, not just purchasing/commissioning. So would be responsible through the RHAs for the integrated providers, and for performance managing and regulating GP services.

In a Health Select Committee report (2010), a review was undertaken on commissioning in England. Central to this area of study is examining the nature of, and the development of, the English NHS internal market. The report is very comprehensive and reviews commissioning structures since 1989, potential weaknesses in commissioning, the effect of wider reforms on commissioning, and how the Government has responded to weaknesses in commissioning. The report also reviewed the potential options for the future.

The report evidence was gathered between October 2009 and February 2010. Essentially the report sought to: understand the costs of commissioning and the purchaser/provider split, and benefits and flaws in the commissioning process

– whilst evaluating options for the future. The Committee looked at options including (a) Abolition of Primary Care Trusts (an earlier manifestation of local commissioning – which were replaced by the Clinical Commissioning Groups (CCGs) following the 2012 Health Act, and then the Integrated Care Boards (ICBs) following the 2022 Act, (b) Keeping PCTs but doing more to integrate care, (c) Retaining PCTs but introducing "local clinical partnerships", (d) Department of Health Commission services, and, (e) Retaining and Strengthening PCTs. The report concluded:

> A number of witnesses argued that we have had the disadvantage of an adversarial system without as yet seeing the benefits from the purchaser/provider split. If reliable figures for the cost of commissioning prove that it is uneconomic and if it does not begin to improve soon, after 20 years of costly failure, the purchaser/provider split may need to be abolished. (Health Select Committee report 2010: 60).

In Allen et al (2020) the approach to commissioning healthcare in England is reviewed. The work reviewed commissioning policy and what it has meant in practice at a time when there was significant flux in the system through the advent of integrated care systems but notes there will be an ongoing role for commissioning (to allocate resources, deliver population health goals and provide provider oversight) irrespective of whether that occurs in a pro-competitive quasi-market or not. In Sheaff (1991, 1995 and 2002) the issues of marketing for healthcare, information systems and the approach to marketing and quality management in the emergent NHS internal market are reviewed respectively, and provide a useful evaluation at points of the evolution of 'Market 1' and 'Market 2'.

The Health Select Committee report (2010), Allen et al (2020), and Sheaff (1991, 1995 and 2002) provide good oversight documents for the development and continuing debate about the quasi-market in the English NHS. Parliament is not the only source of material, however. A further evaluation comes from The Kings' Fund (a charity which seeks to understand how the health system in England can be improved). It aims to work with individuals and organisations to shape policy, transform services and bring about behaviour change. In 2010 the Kings' Fund performed a review of the progress of the NHS in England from 1997 to 2010. The report focussed on trying to establish the level of performance in the NHS in the areas of access to services, patient services, health promotion, clinical effectiveness, patient experience, equity, efficiency and accountability. The report noted that the NHS had made good progress in a number of these areas.

The report identified three different themes in the strategies for NHS reform between 1997 and 2010. The first theme was the support offered to providers, including an increased supply of health professionals, the modernisation of buildings and infrastructure, and support for learning and improvement. The second theme was top-down challenges including targets and national standards, inspection and regulation, publication of performance information, and direct intervention from the centre. The third theme was bottom-up or local challenges, including commissioning, patient choice, and financial incentives such as Payments by Results.

The Kings Fund (2010) report assessed the level of absolute performance along with relative performance against other healthcare systems in other countries. It also tried to look at the improvement in performance over the lifetime of the then-Labour Government but did not attempt to link the evidenced improvements in performance against the reform strategy themes. Without these links, it is difficult to conclude to what extent the various reform levers have individually or combined contributed to the improved performance observed. Perhaps because of, or despite this lack of establishing cause and effect, the report did make some recommendations regarding the future of the NHS and how to improve its performance. The report concludes:

> Finally, even if the relative importance of the NHS goals could be resolved, the question of which levers and mechanisms work best has not yet been explored fully. Since 1997 the government has plotted a number of different courses in relation to harnessing market forces and competition within the NHS. Its first approach was to reject these principles in favour of targets and a regime of tight performance management. Next, it grafted onto this a set of reforms designed to drive improvement through a reformed hospital payment system, financial incentives for NHS organisations and GPs, consumer choice and competition. In the most recent phase, the market style levers are still in place, but ministerial rhetoric has emphasised collaboration, clinical leadership and favouring the NHS over potential independent competitors. These policies have yet to be fully evaluated, and there is little consistent evidence to guide policymakers in the future. (Kings Fund, 2010: 114)

The sheer scale of the reform agenda which is summarized in the Kings Fund report does begin to clearly articulate the challenge for social science research into the English NHS. The breadth and different types of reforms mean that identifying which policy lever has led to a degree of policy success or failure is intrinsically hard to discern. To establish a correlation between them and then develop a theory of causality between them may be impossible.

The "targets and a regime of tight performance management" approach cited in the Health Select Committee report is linked to the idea of 'deliverology' and the emergence of the importance of a potentially invigorated approach to public sector delivery, harnessed following the General Election of 2001. One of the architects of this 'deliverology' approach, Barber (2007: 73) noted:

> There are thousands of people in government bureaucracies whose job it is to complicate matters (lawyers spring to mind – 'It all depends,' they begin). I don't necessarily criticise this – government is, after all, a complicated thing. However, to get anything done, a counter-veiling force is required; people who will simplify, keep bringing people back to the fundamentals:
>
> - What are you trying to do?
> - How are you trying to do it?
> - How do you know you are succeeding?
> - If you're not succeeding, how will you change things?
> - How can we help you?

Mannion, et al (2005) reviewed the nature of cultures for improved performance. The work noted the essential role of understanding organisational culture to deliver performance improvements and how all policy levers need to be appraised of that culture to deliver effectively. Seddon (2008) goes further to debunk the efficacy of targets and choice and market structures in public services as a route to secure their efficient and effective working. He attempts to shape the approach to the public sector based on an analysis of the fundamental motivations of the individuals participating in it, and their need to understand the nature of the value which service users wish and need to derive from the public services they receive. Ultimately, Seddon believes that if the workers in the public sector are regarded as untrustworthy and lazy this will become a self-fulfilling prophecy. This standpoint is one based on his training as an occupational psychologist, who has tried to interpret the Toyota Production System for service organisations. The 'deliverology' approach cannot be criticised in terms of the need to potentially simplify and specify what you are trying to change. However, the problems with this approach, if poorly implemented, can give rise to an overly simplistic set of targets and measures, that do not sensibly, describe the broader outcomes required of complex systems and services.

Seddon's analysis of the health system looks particularly at the area of adult and elderly social care, where his work observed the impact of targets has not necessarily delivered better services. Although Seddon did not focus on the NHS in particular, he began to meet head-on the nature and efficacy of target setting and choice and markets in the arena of public policy. Of interest for this research, therefore, is the extent to which the internal market agenda may be forcing the participants in the system to see the work in a particular way and conform to particular values, and how this may be inhibiting their ability to deliver more value-driven healthcare because of the structures they are working in and through.

Seddon provides a strong antithesis to some of the prevailing NHS managerial approaches regarding target-setting and markets, stressing the importance of systems thinking and practitioner autonomy, which is of interest to the existing NHS policy and management debate. He notes five costs associated with the current regimes, such as that which are in place in the English NHS: (i) the costs of people writing specifications, (ii) the costs of inspection, (iii) the costs of preparing for inspection, (iv) the costs of specifications being wrong, and (v) the costs of demoralization. He proposes a platform for innovation, by changing the locus of control towards innovation, not compliance. He rejects elements of external compliance, focusing on what works and emulating it and having a better view of human nature and proposed that his approach would give rise to significant improvements:

> .... the new architecture liberates public servants from the prison of suspicion and distrust that the current regime locks them into, demeaning their professionalism with simplistic targets and casting them as self-interested producers, as part of the problem. By contrast, the assumptions that I use are no less rational, but they are positive, rather than negative: the new structures assume that people are motivated more by pride in their work than by money, that they are vocational – they want to serve – and that they are capable of using their own ingenuity and initiative. It is also to assume that, in delivering services to consumers and citizens, cooperation will serve our purposes better than competition. People's behaviour is a product of their system. It is only by changing the regime that we can expect a change in behaviour. (Seddon, 2008: 197)

2.6 Further Accounts of the Reasons for and Frailties of the English NHS Market

This chapter will now outline four works which take a more comparative and discursive approach to health policy research and link these views to the development of quasi-market policies. The key works discussed include Greer (2004), Paton (2006), Marmor, (2007) and Fox (2018).

Greer (2004) examines the divergent policies on the health systems in the context of the different approaches to managing healthcare in England, Scotland, Wales and Northern Ireland. This analysis is placed in the context of the devolution of power from the British Parliament to the regional administrations in Wales, Scotland and Northern Ireland which occurred in the Summer of 1999. It could be contended that the United Kingdom healthcare system has become a laboratory for health public policy, by comparing England, Scotland, Wales and Northern Ireland. As HFMA covers all four areas of the UK, this is evident in the discussions which are held on comparative system efficiency and approach through the HFMA Policy and Research Committee.

As a result of devolution, the health systems in the UK have started to diverge in the approach adopted to their management. Greer (2004), like Tuohy (2009), was keen to contextualise the policy arena for health in the UK and states that his research methodology is qualitative. Greer's study was also keen to examine the nature of medical politics and the politics of medicine, to understand the stakeholder perspective of the medical profession within the healthcare system, and the approach to the politics and policy of healthcare within each of the four sub-systems. The role of the different actors in the NHS was examined: from the Secretary of State through the different tiers and roles in the NHS.

Greer's research also provides an account of the wider development of the NHS since its inception in 1948. This looks at the series of NHS reforms which have shaped the development of the system. The reforms in 1974 sought to address issues of decision-making and incorporation of clinicians into the management of the different tiers of the system with a higher degree of integrated professional input. It then noted the development of general management in the system, which was recommended by the Griffiths Report in 1983. The next key development which saw the inception of the internal market was also described starting with the initial quasi-market in 1989. It also described the quasi-market period under New Labour from 1998.

Greer categorised each of the four UK health systems with their own brand of NHS approach. The Scottish approach to the management of the NHS was said to be described as 'professionalism', which was defined by breaking from the market mechanisms of England, due to policies gaining acceptance which were politically to the left of those in England, and due to the interplay between the Scottish political institutions and the senior employees of the NHS in Scotland, particularly the medics. The English NHS was said to be described by 'markets', although this term is somewhat complicated. The rationalisation of this from a political perspective was identified as the political centre-ground in England is more right-wing than the political consensus in Scotland or Wales. The policy in Wales was defined by 'localism', in that there seems to be a higher degree of trust in public services themselves. Whereas Northern Irish politics has been focussed elsewhere during the development of healthcare public policy. Healthcare policy in Northern Ireland was defined as "permissive managerialism", seeking to run the system with a minimum of fuss to deliver the required outcomes. Although noting the differences in the four systems, the Greer study does not make claims on their relative efficacy but bases its descriptions of the UK subsystems on the political and institutional factors in play that described the approaches leading to their formation.

Paton (2006) examined the interplay between health, public policy and politics. This account overtly centres health policy in a political context. It asserted that the quasi-market in the English NHS was a function of New Labour's need to try and identify a radical agenda, and as a way for the senior figures in the party to reconcile the health system to global capitalism and EU competition regulation. Also, for the publicly funded system to demonstrate its effectiveness, when compared with other potential funding and provision systems for health, the English NHS system with the internal market may have demonstrated some need for efficiency, which appealed to a more right-of-centre Downsian median voter in England. Downs (1957) described the median voter as the middle of a left/right political continuum. The English MPs in Parliament always tend to have a higher proportion of Conservatives, than for those in Wales, or Scotland (ignoring the complexity of the unionist/ republican divide in Northern Ireland).

Paton went on to identify some core issues within the policy environment which seemed to be contradictory regarding (a) whether the Primary Care Trust (PCT) – one of the earlier incarnations of the commissioning bodies – structure represented devolution of power or just increased transaction costs; (b) if we truly had patient choice what was the role for a tier of administration doing purchasing or commissioning; (c) if we had a market why were exhortations to collaborate necessary; and (d) if the market was effective why were so many nationally determined targets seemingly necessary.

Paton was clear in articulating the policy tensions in the NHS systems that existed from 1997 to 2010. It articulated the key policy tensions in the health public policy arena, concerning trust in the practitioners who work within the systems themselves, and their propensity for altruistic 'Knightly" behaviour, or the need to closely monitor their progress, because of their potential inability to work to the common good, as 'Knaves'. Le Grand (2003: 45) had previously described the need to be concerned with the motivations of those in the public sector to help design public policy: 'The term "knave" is used to mean simply an individual whose principal concern is to further his or her self-interest.'

The definition of 'knights' was seen by Le Grand as more problematic, but centred on the concept of moral, collectivist, public-spirited or pro-social and altruistic behaviours. A core difficulty in public policy results from the need to determine the motivations of those within it. It is perhaps this tension that has resulted in a lack of clarity in the delivery of public policy, and the need for an emergent and controlling bureaucracy, as identified by Paton (2006: 150):

> The new bureaucracy has been a major theme of the new Labour state [created up to 2006]. Schools, universities and health ... increasingly choice and market rhetoric; increasingly bureaucratic reality.

Marmor (2007) reviewed the problems of simplistically applying management theory or public policy 'initiative' approaches to healthcare. He also saw the difficulties of transnational policy adoption to improve services. He examined the evidence of an international trend towards the adoption of more business-like and market-orientated language in health policy. On reviewing the NHS, Marmor developed a summary of the ideas used to describe the New Public Management prevalent in the extant public policy in health, which:

> ...consists of a cluster of ideas borrowed from the conceptual framework of private sector management. Among the ideas most emphasised are i) cost control, financial transparency, and decentralisation of management authority; ii) the creation of market and quasi-market mechanisms separating purchasing from providing functions and their linkage via contracts; and, iii) the enhancement of accountability to customers for the quality of their service via the creation of performance indicators. (Marmor, 2007:15)

These ideas, from an existing health service management practitioner perspective, continue to be prevalent within the NHS currently; and it is important to review the extent to which they have challenged the previous orthodoxy of the role of doctors and (their) administrators, in previous incarnations of the NHS health system, particularly prior to 1974. Perhaps, the area discussed by Marmor which impacts heavily on the intended area of this practitioner's thesis is the area of targets and their centralising consequence, which is also referred to in Paton's work. Most particularly, these studies provide a conceptual framework in which to ground a thesis on quasi-markets, by looking at the policy, its development and implementation, and the underpinning rationale behind it.

A further consideration which needs to be given to any proposed renewal of the current NHS structure probably also needs to fundamentally address the role of the state versus the citizen:

> In the health and care sectors, there is a wide consensus on the need to keep people from arriving at the hospital gates and other forms of institutional care. But while ideas of prevention and early intervention are based on the belief that the boundaries can be redrawn, not erased, they themselves rest on familiar assumptions about the divide between community-based citizens and the subjects of service land, rather than removing the divide. (Fox (2018); 3)

Fox (2018) wrote based on his experience in the social care sector and sought to better express the need for an enhanced role in health and well-being for the voluntary, community and social enterprise sectors. Fox based his analysis on a belief in the role of voluntary and community action and the fundamental belief that health and care services need to be much more closely integrated with the needs and wishes of the communities and citizens that the system serves. He noted that this work has been underway in the local government social care sector but has not really taken hold in healthcare or been utilised in healthcare.

> England's adult social care system has seen one of the most concerted and long-standing attempts at radical reform of a national public service in the Western world. Called 'personalisation', a term that never gained widespread understanding, it could be described as the attempt to 'humanise' the long-term support of disabled adults and to a lesser extent, older people. (Fox,2018: 87).

One of the key issues with the delivery of health care is the different funding mechanisms associated with it. For example, health services are free at the point of need, versus care services which are based on the ability to pay, with some care funded by the individual or local government agencies, based on their ability to pay. Social Care provision is particularly problematic when family structures step in to provide the care. Once individuals are coping, without further support, it is then necessary to evidence when the family or support network can no longer cope, and why the situation has changed before local government funding can begin.

The relationship between self-care, community-based care and the care given by the state through the NHS is difficult to describe (and often prescribe) but will become increasingly important as demographic changes lead to a further ageing population, and changing technology becomes available, to help citizens manage their own conditions. Here there will need to be a clarification of the role of self-care and the duty of care which the medical profession and wider health service need to deliver. The power of the citizens to deliver their own care could be a force to be reckoned with:

The NHS in England has appointed three organisations in 2016, the New Economics Foundation, Nesta and the Royal Society of Arts, to lead a programme called Health as a Social Movement. Its first report (Del Castillo et al, 2016) notes how extraordinary it is for a major public sector leader, NHS England Chief Executive Simon Stevens, actively to call for social movements within his domain, given that social movements, are by their very nature grassroots, messy and keen to challenge those in power. (Fox, 2018: 171)

The internal market structure may be seen as an impediment to the sort of care integration that may enable community engagement in care, and more seamless pathways in and out of care in a more acute setting, such as hospitals. Indeed, without a changed structure, such as that suggested by Paton the very rigid structures and separations in healthcare may be seen to work against that integration and citizen empowerment aim. It is for these reasons, that following the 2012 Act, NHS England (and NHS Improvement) sought to introduce new sorts of structures into the English NHS. The originally titled Sustainability and Transformation Plans sought to develop intermediate structures to allow a common planning framework with an equal voice for commissioners, providers and local government, in a locally determined geography, covering between a circa 400,000 to 2.5m population. There were 42 STPs in England, one for Derbyshire, where the author was the finance lead. These were seen as a potential vehicle for reducing the barriers to delivering a more integrated health and care service. The House of Commons - Health Committee (2018) report on Integrated Care sought to further these aims and recommended:

a) Develop a national transformation strategy backed by secure long-term funding to support local areas to accelerate progress towards more collaborative, place-based and integrated care.

b) Commit to a dedicated, ring-fenced transformation fund.

c) Explain the case for change clearly and persuasively, including why it matters to join up care for the benefit of the patients and the public.

d) Alongside these changes, the Government should facilitate the national bodies to work with representatives from across the health and care community who should lead in bringing forward legislative proposals to overcome the current fragmentation and legal barriers arising out of the Health and Social Care Act 2012. These proposals should be laid before the House in draft and presented to us for pre-legislative scrutiny.

[Legislative change was proposed, including]:

- A statutory basis for system-wide partnerships between organisations.
- Potentially to designate Accountable Care Organisations (ACOs) as NHS bodies, if they are introduced more widely.
- Changes to legislation covering procurement and competition.
- The merger of NHS England and NHS Improvement; and
- CQC regulatory powers. (House of Commons - Health Committee, 2018: 6)

There was, therefore, a cross-party and growing consensus that the internal market structure had had its day, and structures are being put in place, supported by the 2022 Act, to enable a change in how the NHS is run, which is described in The NHS Long Term Plan. Also, there was a good deal of academic and wider literature explaining the frailties and downsides of the internal market structure

2.7 Theories of Public Policy Implementation

The approach to studying public policy implementation is varied and there is academic public policy literature on implementation. The author is interested in the finance practitioner role within the English NHS, and the practitioner role in implementing and delivering policy. Sabatier and Mamanian (1983: 540) defined implementation as:

> …the carrying out of a basic policy decision, usually made in a statute (although also possible through important executive orders or court decisions). Ideally, that decision identifies the problem(s) to be addressed, stipulates the objective(s) to be pursued, and in a variety of ways, "structures" the implementation process.

If one starts to critically appraise Market 1, Market 2 or Market 3 against this implementation and public policy definition it is possible to ascertain the basic policy decision, the objectives to be pursued and the way in which the implementation is structured. Market 1, particularly in "Working for Patients", challenged the old order of the English NHS and described different structures for implementation, via new organisations, with revised objectives. What has been slightly less clear is the extent to which the policy, the implementation of the policy, or the feedback and interaction from the stakeholders in the policy, go on to describe the success or failure of the policy itself. Sabatier and Mazmanian (1983: 554) noted:

> ...successful implementation in the short run is especially dependent upon the strength of the statute, particularly the degree of hierarchical integration, the commitment of agency officials, the presence of a "fixer" and the resources of various constituency groups. In the long run, however, it is the changing socio-economic conditions and the ability of supportive constituency groups to effectively intervene in the process that are probably the most important.

Sabatier and Mazmanian noted that the immediate success of implementation would tend to be defined by the clarity of the policy and the ease with which officials can instruct and get on with implementing. In the context of the NHS internal market the clarity with which the "constituency groups", such as NHS finance practitioners, approved of and therefore have supported the policy is a large determinant of longer-term potential success. In the medium term this clarity, ease and instruction tend to get more de-railed or supported by the feedback from the system participants themselves. The author wishes therefore to determine the level of support for the policy, within his own finance practitioner epistemic group. A similar analysis of the ease of implementation was also given in a seminal work on implementation by Pressman and Wildavsky (1973: 147):

> Experience with the innumerable steps involved in programme implementation suggest that simplicity in policies is much to be desired. The fewer steps involved in carrying out the programme, the fewer the opportunities for a disaster to overtake it. The more directly the policy aims at its target, the fewer the decisions involved in its ultimate realisation and the greater the likelihood of implementation.

It is somewhat intuitive that the simpler the policy, the easier the level of control in the system and the absence of practitioner resistance in the medium term, the more embedded and successful the policy is likely to become, with an alignment between policy goals and those charged with delivering policy. In the context of the NHS internal market, these criteria are interesting to reflect upon. Essentially, if the policy is complicated, the nature of the delivery of healthcare is multi-faceted, and the environment in which the policy is implemented has different institutional dimensions, and if there are different organisations to be influenced and controlled which have different complex institutional and structural dimensions, this makes the policy implementation process complex and fraught. Given this complexity, the likelihood of policy success is likely to be low. Because of these factors Ham (2009: 231) noted:

> Policymaking in NHS bodies involves a range of interests each seeking to influence what is decided. In assessing the strength of

these agencies and interests, the powerful position occupied by the medical profession is again apparent. Although governments have taken action to make doctors more accountable, as in the changes . . . introduced by the Blair government . . . speaks volumes about the ability of the profession to delay to resist policies that threaten clinical autonomy.

In addition to the impact of the medical profession, and other professional groups within the NHS, there is also the influence of other policies within the NHS impacting upon the internal market. As a consequence of this Ham (2009: 239) goes on to further describe:

> Continuing reliance on hierarchical controls is reinforced by the disappointing effects of markets as a tool for healthcare reform. In two publications, Le Grand has made the case for markets by reference to the motivations of the providers of public services ...Specifically, he argues that providers exhibit both knightly and knavish behaviours and that public service reform cannot rely on the assumption that providers are essentially altruistic individuals who are committed to delivering high-quality services to users. Rather, Le Grand contends that quasi markets are needed to counteract the risk of self-interested behaviours by providers, the bias towards the middle classes that arise when reforms depend on users exercising voice and disempowerment that results from overreliance on hierarchical controls.

Given that Le Grand was once a special advisor to the Department of Health and advised on the implementation of the quasi-market to the Blair administration, through the Prime Minister's Delivery Unit, this is probably one of the clearest rationales for the internal Market 2 that is available to the researcher. The fact that the Government of the day did not identify the 'knavish' behaviour of the producer interest, in the NHS, is hardly surprising given that this motivation for reform has a high degree of negative connotation for the NHS, which is normally held in high esteem by the electorate in England. Much public opinion polling in recent years tended to show the NHS as a well-regarded institution. It could therefore be argued, that the high esteem in which the NHS is held, meant the rationale for the internal-market policy reforms, challenging the NHS producer interest, itself, was not the stated reason. This may be why that rationale was suppressed from the public policy rationale.

To understand if the market in the English NHS could be a success, it is important to understand the funding mechanism within the system. A detailed understanding of the delivery mechanism of the quasi-market is necessary to appraise success. Since 'Working for Patients' the reimbursement mechanism in the English hospital sector has been the activity performed by the hospital. Although this payment system (Payment by Results) has been reformed and changed during this period, it may, at this point it may be worth questioning whether the initial aim of the system was to purely move from cash to volume budgeting, as opposed to the commencement of a market. This would see the initial and probably sensible objective of Market 1 as a move towards a changed funding formula for hospitals not based on historical budgets but based on the level of clinical activity performed. This type of budgeting was described by Wildavsky (1992: 432):

> Budgeting can be done not only in cash but also in terms of volume. Instead of promising to pay so much over the next year or years, the commitment can be made in terms of operations to be performed or services provided.

When appraising the development of the public policy on quasi-markets, it is important to bear in mind the fact that there have been multiple policy objectives, at particular phases of the policy under development. A key objective of Market 1, therefore, was overtly to move from cash to volume budgeting to incentivise hospitals to reduce long waiting times. A plural provider marketplace with choice in healthcare providers was more of an overt objective for Market 2. Given the potential dissonance between the stated aims of Market 2 and the "knavish" description of Le Grand, it can be difficult to identify the absolute policy goals. The fundamental aims of Market 3 were probably to give an improved structure and instruments to enable the original policy objectives of Market 1 and Market 2 to be more successful.

Public policy analysis offers useful insights which can be used in studying health policy and management. For example, John (1998) identified two broad areas in which public policy scholars can operate (i) policy variation between sectors such as health and education and/or between countries, and (ii) policy change, how do policies become stable? And why do policies emerge and/or fall out of favour? Public policy analysis offers several relevant approaches to analysis – institutional, group/network, socio-economic, rational choice, and ideation. For this research, the author was interested in the role of 'ideas' that generated the stated or implicit aims of the internal market. Ideational analysis focuses on the role of ideas as solutions to policy problems, and they are claimed to have a life of their own (Kingdon, 1995). Ideas circulate and gain influence independently or prior to the interests of the policy process. But the research is also interested in how institutions and groups/networks have maintained this policy, beyond the point at which many commentators/actors have started to assert that there is a need for a change in approach and structure. In trying to draw conclusions on the extent to which public policy is delivering the desired aims for the policy there is an approach to trying to appraise policy through implementation studies. Hill and Hupe (2002: 200) noted:

> ... implementation is a complex matter. This recognition came to scholars as they moved away from the early arguments about the subject, at just the same time as the complexities of governance as opposed to government were being recognized. As such it is neither easy to research nor easy to influence. In the face of such recognition one way forward is the pessimistic route of saying it is all too difficult; researchers therefore can only describe what happens and policy actors can only operate intuitively. The alternative is to recognize processes that can be understood by research and influenced by policy actors, in a context in which there is much that is both intriguing to understand and worthwhile to control. This is the alternative we advocate.

Baggot (2007) gave us a series of conceptual frameworks to potentially evaluate health policy. They included, (i) policy as a rational, hierarchical process (there is a policy that emanates from higher up in a structure), (ii) policy, ideology and political parties (there is an interplay between ideas/concepts, political policies and public policy), (iii) policy as an interplay of interests (pressure group roles and opinions and objectives are central to this analysis), (iv) policy institutions and agendas (puts the institutions themselves as important players in the policy process), and (v) policy as an adaptive learning process (notes the importance of networks and coalitions to develop and implement policy). For this study, the author is not persuaded that the NHS internal market policy as a rational, hierarchal process quite fits. The reasons for the policy were never clearly stated. There is an ideological standpoint in markets, but institutions and the role of interests in those institutions and their agendas seem to have helped with the perpetuation of the internal market policies:

> Applying the concept of policy networks to health policy facilitates mapping of a range of government and non-government organisations involved in the policy arena. It is also useful around posing questions about how the changing relationships between government and groups might affect policy formation, implementation and outcomes. Indeed, it appears that the tightly knit 'policy community' that characterised the immediate post-war period, exemplified by the close relationship between the BMA and the Ministry for Health, has given way to a looser, more inclusive 'issue network'. (Baggot, 2007: 11)

2.8 Top Down and Bottom-Up Approaches to Policy Implementation, the Role of Epistemic Groups and the Advocacy Coalition Framework

The complexity of the NHS internal market policy is apparent and how it is influenced is somewhat opaque. There is a policy framework which has evolved over a considerable period, the objectives and originating reasons for that policy are contested and there are an array of actors and organisations which are then influenced by and trying to adopt or adapt that policy, or not. Hill (2005: 227) described:

> The British National Health Service (NHS) has experienced turbulent, top-down-driven change through most of its history, and certainly since the later 1980s. Issues about striving for top-down control have been much in evidence, contracting (the transaction mode) has been tried and largely (but not entirely) discarded, and a great deal of attention has been paid to ways of steering the work of professional staff.

Two different schools of implementation analysis are associated with public policy: top-down and bottom-up. The first top-down approach, to reviewing implementation is to review the policy framework and coherence and policy adoption at the state or macro level. The second is to review the policy adoption at the implementation level. The former analysis is perhaps most appropriate if there is coherence within the coalitions which tend to set the policy framework. In reviewing where the policy study is best aimed, Matland (1995: 170) observed:

> Traditional top-down models, based on the public administration tradition, present an accurate description of the implementation process where the policy is clear and the conflict is low…Because there is a clear policy, macro-implementation planners wield considerable influence. Bottom-up models provide an accurate description when policy is ambiguous and conflict is low…When there is substantial conflict and ambiguous policy, both models have some relevancy.

The policy underpinning of the NHS market reform may be traced back to a New Right view on public sector efficacy versus market efficacy. Once that notion is understood, the top-down policy driver for the NHS market can be understood. In determining whether the policy itself is good, it is also necessary to critically appraise the healthcare sector as an environment where market mechanisms can effectively function; and appraise what other factors could be influencing that. Without isolating these factors, it is not possible to appraise the market policy.

The extent to which the policy was successfully adopted, once this market approach was understood, requires an appraisal based on the bottom-up adoption practices at the practitioner level within the NHS system itself. Analysis of this is possible, and a study by May and Winter appraised the factors which give rise to successful implementation, in the specific context of labour reform in Denmark, but with a result that could be generalised. They essentially concluded policy implementation needs practitioner understanding and approval for adoption as described by May and Winter (2007: 469):

> . . . our findings provide a more nuanced and positive assessment than much of the implementation literature of the way that higher-level policies are translated into action at the frontlines. . . The signalling of policy goals by elected municipal elected officials and managerial actions of employment services managers are relevant, but these factors seem to have limited influence. More important is the understanding of the national policy by street-level bureaucrats and their knowledge of the rules under the reform.

The practitioner understanding amongst the groups of those delivering policy is, therefore, an important factor in deriving the success of the policy. Evaluating the nature and extent of policy success is a useful concept for this thesis. McConnell (2010) identifies six important strands in the evaluation of policy success or failure which are i) societal benefit, ii) public value, iii) good practice in policymaking and development, iv) how policy accrues benefits to political actors, v) explicitly acknowledges that policy success is likely to only be marginal, vi) the fact that policy avoids absolute failure or fiasco. He then goes on to classify policy a) process, b) programme/delivery and c) politics as either a resilient success, conflicted success, precarious success or a failure. This may be a useful framework to review the extent to which the internal market has been a success or failure, noting that an absolute determination in these different dimensions is exceptionally hard. McConnell's (2010: 346) core definition of policy success is "if it achieves the goals that proposed set out to achieve and attract no criticism of any significance and or support is virtually universal".

McConnell then goes on to describe contradictions between different forms of success, whereby it is possible to have a successful process but unsuccessful programme/outcomes. It is also possible to be politically successful with policy but have an unsuccessful programme/outcome. Also, it is possible to have a successful programme which delivers outcomes but has unsuccessful politics. These different outcomes will be explored in the conclusions of the thesis.

In the current and previous structures, the author has operated in, in the English NHS, a key issue explored through the thesis is the role of practitioners in both influencing the implementation of policy and the policy itself. Lipsky explored this concept through the idea of "street-level bureaucrats", who do not develop policy but can help or hinder its delivery. Lipsky (2010: 13) noted:

> Street-level bureaucrats make policy in two related respects. They exercise wide discretion in decisions about the citizens with whom they interact. Then, when taken in concert, their individual actions add up to agency behaviour... the position of street-level bureaucrats regularly permits them to make policy with respect to their interactions with citizens.

The approach and role of practitioners in NHS finance warrant a discussion of their status and role. To what extent are they acting to "mediate between science and society to translate scientific research into social progress" as described by Schon (1983), maybe a debate about the extent to which the NHS finance profession is an epistemic community. Epistemic communities were defined by Dunlop (2013) as:

> ....groups of professionals, often from a variety of different disciplines, which produce policy-relevant knowledge about complex technical issues...Such communities embody a belief system around an issue which contains four knowledge elements: 1) a shared set of normative and principled beliefs. . . ; 2) shared causal beliefs, which are derived from their analysis of practices . . . ; 3) shared notions of validity – that is, intersubjective, . . . and 4) a common policy enterprise – that is, a set of common practices... (Dunlop, 2013: 229).

The extent to which either NHS finance practitioners, HFMA or CIPFA represent this type of epistemic community, with a shared set of (1) beliefs, (2) causal understandings ideas, (3) views on validity and (4) a common enterprise, will be discussed and questioned later in this work. It is possible that NHS finance practitioners are both an epistemic community and "street-level bureaucrats" and can choose which way they wish to behave towards policy adoption. CIPFA and HFMA have a role to help represent these views and try and advocate for them.

Dissatisfaction with the competing top-down and bottom-up approach to studying policy and the need to regard the actors in the policy process as central in themselves saw the development of the Advocacy Coalition Framework (ACF). This seeks to explain the development, endurance and longevity of policy via a more detailed study of the coalitions of actors for and around particular policy and seeking to understand consensus, patterns of co-ordination, looking at how policy goals are met via an understanding of how coalitions form, remain stable and negotiate with opponents. This model therefore specifically seeks to understand the role and coherence of epistemic groups around policy, as described by Weible (2013: 125):

> Sabatier and Jenkins-Smith established the ACF in response to several perceived shortcomings in policy process research: a dissatisfaction with the policy cycle or stages heuristic as a causal theory; a need to take more seriously the role of scientific and technical information in policy processes; dissatisfaction with the top-down and bottom-up perspectives of the implementation literature; a need to take a long-term time perspective to understand policy processes; and a need to develop theories that assume more realistic human agents other than the rational actor models found in microeconomics.

The author's research on NHS market reform practitioner views and how the reforms are reviewed, as well as on the policy underpinning the efficacy of market mechanisms, is therefore important. A further factor that is impacting the policy environment within the English NHS is the state institutional dimension of hierarchy and control. Whilst the market has been developed in the English NHS, there has also been a large policy strand around targets and managerialism. The efficacy of these targets has also been critically appraised by academics in policy implementation. For example, the star system was a rating mechanism using key targets for hospitals at the time of Market 2, which has largely remained unchanged since. Bevan and Hood (2006: 553) noted:

> We see the system of star rating as a process of 'learning by doing' in which the Government chose to ignore the problems we have identified. A consequence was that although there were indeed dramatic improvements in reported performance, we do not know the extent to which these were genuine or offset by gaming that resulted in reductions in performance that were not captured by targets. Evidence of gaming naturally led many critics of New Labour's targets-and-terror regime to advocate the wholesale abandonment of that system... Nor is health care truly governed by anything approximating to a free market in any developed state: regulation and public funding (even in the form of tax expenditures) take centre stage in every case.

When trying to determine policy success therefore which is already contested, as noted above, a further complication in the English NHS surrounds which particular policy was creating an effect within the service. Also, with some of the policies, such as with the star rating system, there may have been further issues associated with poor outcomes, either associated with the policy itself, or with the measures of the policy success, creating unintended consequences, as noted by Bevan and Hood (2006) and Seddon (2008). A further study on the role of targets in public policy by Schofield and Sausman (2004: 245) noted:

> One of the consequences for policy implementation of corporate public governance organised via a system of assurance is the danger of implementing policy for compliance means only. This can be described as compliance with the required audit tools, rather than for the solution of the policy problem. What happens then is a form of regulatory capture, thus 'what counts becomes what matters,' rather than, 'what matters counts'. The accountability system that follows this is more likely to measure output than outcome . . . Under such a system, questions about implementation become questions about compliance and performance rather than problem-solving.

Barrett (2004) forms similar conclusions on the role of targets and compliance in the English public policy arena. She specifically also argues that studies of the implementation and change process are required in this context due to the need to understand the dynamic process of policy implementation:

> There is still a lack of attention in the process in governance theory and practice, in particular explicit attention to the appropriateness of differing conceptualisations of the policy-action relationship to desired outcomes (means and ends). What are the relative benefits of negotiation/learning strategies versus more coercive strategies in differing policy environments? The understanding of the process is also an essential part of capacity building addressing questions such as: Is this doable? How might it work? What would it take? (Barrett, 2004; 260).

From the literature examined, it is clear to the author that there are issues in assessing the policy of the market in isolation. There is at least one further policy implementation variable of 'targets', and the question concerning the coherence of the market policy. The market policy could be appraised on a top-down or bottom-up basis. There is also the complication of the policy implementation being a process not an enactment of solely good or bad policy objectives. The extent to which the current NHS system practitioner opinion is positive or negative on the current structures is hugely significant, in the author's opinion. If the bottom-up, street-level bureaucrats' view of the policy is negative what does that then mean for the English NHS? Should the policy be changed based on that? Also, to what extent is there a need for a major change in the policy direction, or the statute law that governs the system, and to what extent the policy is failing on a; a) process, b) programme or c) political level?

It can further be noted that there is also the factor of the 'collegiate approach' of clinicians, and wider participants, in the healthcare system, perhaps embodied by the Health Act 2012 'duty to co-operate', post 'Pause' amendment. This marks a third strand of the policy environment, in addition to the target and market policy strands in operation, described above. There is probably a contradiction between these policy strands (market and cooperation), and perhaps also the first (targets). Moran (2002: 404) described the idea of the 'regulatory state':

> The study of the regulatory state in Britain is inseparable from the convulsions that came over the British government in the last two decades of the twentieth century, notably those associated with the most ambitious programme of privatisation in the advanced capitalist world and the changes in the workings of central government sometimes summarised as the 'New Public Management'.

In summarising his position on his international review of the regulatory state Moran noted three conclusions: (1) it is a fiction, (2) it exists but is dependent on national setting (he noted in this area that "the British regulatory state is emblematic of the famed contradictions of Thatcherism, simultaneously involving an attempt to dismantle and to centralise state controls)," or (3) the regulatory state is part of a new governing paradigm where governing became governance, a matter of steering networks rather than setting absolute direction.

This wider socio-economic narrative from Moran also exposed a key risk to the researcher in English NHS health policy, in that there may well be an innate policy tension between state regulation and marketisation that makes the policy environment inherently incoherent. Despite the policy tensions and political backdrop of government control and marketisation, there is a need to be able to sensibly evaluate policy, despite its different conception strands and therefore intents and complexity.

2.9 Literature Review Conclusions

There was a political consensus on the state provision of the NHS from 1948 to 1979. This also included a Health Act in 1974 which sought to further unify the provision structures. From 1979 onwards, however, and the Thatcher Administration, initially, there has been an increasing challenge to the state provision of the English NHS, which resulted in an internal market mechanism and a separation between commissioning organisations and provider organisations. This split, however, did not unify provision through primary care, community care and social care and has resulted in several issues associated with the effective delivery of care and an inefficient market.

In addition, several accounts of the market approach have noted the contention around the precise reasons for the development of, and the reality of, the policy. We could therefore suggest there has been a lack of policy coherence, which may have resulted in a lack of successful implementation, either because the policy itself was unclear, or the policy itself was not welcomed by the participants in the system, or the fact that the policy landscape had several competing strands of policy to try and improve the performance of the English NHS during this time.

Given the complexity of the policy environment, and the lack of a political, academic and practitioner consensus on the nature and efficacy of NHS market policy it is perhaps unsurprising that such divergent views arise. The author wishes to attempt to fill some of this divergent gap, with the secondary analysis of the statutory data on hospital (and healthcare organisation) finances and their relative performance; and, with the following attitudinal research on practitioners' views. These two research areas seek to understand the interaction between policy and practice observed by Barrett (2004). Of interest, in the third research phase, was the need to understand the views of different stakeholders on the role and importance of the three institutional dimensions acting in the NHS; markets, targets and cooperation.

Since the 2012 Act, however, there have been rapid changes and non-statutory moves away from the market, through Sustainability and Transformation Plans and then the further development of policy through the Long-Term Plan towards Integrated Care Systems. These have been supported further by the 2022 Act. Despite these moves, however, the statutory organisations are still geared up to deliver a purchaser/provider split, and the potential fractures to policy delivery continue (the purchaser/provider split itself and the separation between DHSC and DLUHC) as identified in Chapter 1.

The next chapter will review the methodology to further research the internal market policy and the approach adopted to answer the three research questions. Chapter 4 will review the extent to which the pricing, and funding, mechanism for health services could ever have been sophisticated enough, irrespective of its desirability, to deliver an internal market in healthcare. Chapter 5 will look at finance practitioner views - on the internal market structure to establish the current and previous appetite for - those working in the system to deliver an internal market. Then, Chapter 6 will review the role of NHS finance practitioners in adopting, adapting and influencing policy.

CHAPTER 3

METHODOLOGY: POSITIONALITY AND PRACTITIONERR RESEARCH

This chapter describes the research methods selected for this thesis and why they were chosen. It describes how the design of the research methodology has changed through the course of the study, and the way this has been informed by the changing role of the author and his levels of access to information and individuals. Also, it describes how the role of the author, and the research design are interrelated. It reviews approaches to practitioner research, the nature of action research, and how the research is informed by the author's ambition to both explain the origins of the NHS internal market, and influence and change it through this research and his roles.

3.1 Practitioner Research and the Evolving Role of this Practitioner

The author has worked in the NHS since 1993 and has held several posts in NHS Finance for nearly thirty years. This has predominantly been within the hospital sector, but the author has also held posts working closer with the DoH, both with the Trust Development Authority (TDA) and then NHS Improvement (NHSI). The author is now in a relatively new role as the Chief Finance Officer of the South Yorkshire Integrated Care Board; formerly he was Director of Finance at Derby Hospitals for eight years.

The original motivation for the development of this thesis was in response to the clamour, at the time, which continues today, for "evidence-based medicine" as described via a BMJ article by Sackett et al (1996). During his career, the author has been interested in the equivalent idea of evidence-based public policy and evidence-based management. During the ongoing development of the internal market there seemed little evidence that it would lead to greater allocative or wider efficiency in health and that there might be unintended and negative consequences of implementing or continuing with the policy.

One of the problems for social science, particularly perhaps, in the public policy environment is seeing whether a common understanding of the causalities or events exists as described in Chapter 2. To make positive claims on the need for changes in structures or funding mechanisms, it is important to ascertain whether there is a well-understood or acknowledged common description of the phenomenon, or policy environment, in question. There can, for example, be several explanations for the NHS including both descriptions of who was involved and how things were done. Powell (2012: 55) reviewed different studies from different perspectives and times on the creation of the NHS, and there is scope for contested interpretations of NHS policy to continue:

> It is difficult to dispute that the creation of the NHS is significant. It is less clear whether the accounts are complete. The early accounts do not display sufficient evidence and are incomplete because they lacked access to the archives . . . To some extent, some different conclusions are available to later writers . . . studies on its creation exhibit 'mixed messages, diverse interpretations', illustrating the 'contested interpretation of historical interpretation'.

Practitioner Research, when compared with 'purer' academic research can suffer from the accusation of bias, a challenge throughout this thesis, as described by Drake and Heath (2011: 19):

> The relationship between the doctoral study and the professional setting raises several important issues for practitioner-researchers, with the most important being the question of whether 'insiders' can achieve any meaningful degree of critical distance from their workplace or their colleagues. But it is the development of this critical position with respect to research and the research setting that defines doctoral-level study.

There is, therefore, a tension within this work, that will be described further in this chapter - regarding (a) the access allowed by the author's role to data and individuals, and (b) the degree of neutrality which can be brought to that role and access, and (c) whether it is possible to reach unbiassed and valid perspectives and conclusions, in that context.

Different perspectives can be used in health and health policy research. There are relative merits and demerits of positive versus anti-positive or normative research. Policy implementation, particularly focussing on the NHS in England, and the development and adoption of quasi-market policies have a range of different interpretations and perspectives. Also, the interaction between the development of these quasi-market policies and the growing managerialism in the public sector, as defined using targets is of interest. The interrelationships between these different elements make positive conclusions on specific policy success or failure hard.

Bowling (2009) provided an overview of the different approaches to health and health service research. The competing and complementary approaches are many and varied. Health service research can very much be a multidisciplinary activity, including several academic disciplines. However, a phenomenological challenge exists here, as definitions of health itself are somewhat problematic, and therefore the efficacy of health policy can be similarly difficult to define.

> Social scientists distinguish between the medical concept of disease, and the subjective feelings and perceptions of disease, often labelled as illness or sickness by lay people. Illness and sickness, unlike disease, are not necessarily detected by biochemical indicators. Research shows that some people can be diseased according to biochemical indicators, without actually feeling sick or ill (e.g., high blood pressure), and others can feel ill without any biochemical evidence of being diseased (e.g. chronic back pain). Health and ill health are viewed by social scientists as a continuum along which individuals progress and regress. (Bowling, 2009: 21)

Even though "health" may be hard to describe and define, this should nevertheless be possible, but the broader definition of "triple value healthcare" (Gray: 2017) contains elements of subjectivity. Despite this, we do have a generalised societal understanding of health and healthcare. There is, therefore, scope for health research to adopt a positive and empirical approach to research, as undertaken by epidemiologists and health economists, alongside potentially more anti-positive perspectives, from political science and management science. For this thesis, there is an assumed definition of health policy, which seeks to raise the standard of health and well-being via policy that positively impacts the health of the English population and best enables improvement. Although as noted in chapter 1, the precise policy aims of the English NHS between, i) efficiency, ii) equity, iii) effectiveness, v) best outcomes, and vi) reducing health inequalities are unclear and overlapping.

The methodology used to evaluate the market system needs to be mindful of the Le Grand (2003) 'Knightly' and 'Knavish' dichotomy, described by Seddon (2008) and Barber (2007), respectively. As the main motivation here for undertaking doctoral, practitioner-based, research in health is to evaluate the evidence for the market approach, this tension is centre-stage. There also needs to be good policy and good implementation, to make the policy effective, to ultimately improve the health and well-being of the population. There are varied approaches around the NHS that on occasion may be seen as competing, as opposed to complementary approaches (e.g., systems thinking, and delivery might be difficult in the internal market structure). Exworthy et al (2023) analysed approaches to governing the English NHS through hierarchies, markets and networks, described through three different axes: 1) public and private; 2) centralisation and decentralisation, and 3) professional and state. Building on this, this author identifies five different reform approaches to the management of the English NHS:

i. quasi-market reform – building the approach to an internal market mimicking the private sector, started in the English NHS By Working for Patients (1989).

ii. target setting – centralising control and managing through top-down targets building on the work by Barber (2007).

iii. fundamental systems thinking – allowing decentralisation and professional control described by Seddon (2008).

iv. improved management approaches – perhaps initiated by Griffiths (1983) in the English NHS.

v. other and wider public policy initiatives – there are many other approaches to trying to deliver improved policies that will impact on health.

These five different reform approaches are not paradigms with one about to win out to become the prevailing and complete public policy orthodoxy, in the English NHS, but the different approaches need acknowledgement. Also, the research needs to be very mindful of their existence. They describe differently the actions of those in the public sector, and those who try and control them, and they also potentially describe different motivations for the groups within and around these systems. The theoretical underpinning of good policy and practice would seemingly need to reconcile or discount some of these views or align them, to provide an underlying framework for describing a robust approach to public policy determination and improving health and care outcomes.

In selecting a practitioner research methodology, the author has chosen different debates in health policy and practice, to be explored as part of the thesis topic regarding the reform agenda inside the English NHS. It is hard to separate this analysis from the author's own beliefs and opinions on the development of NHS policy, which is unsurprising given that this is the arena in which the author works. It is also unsurprising that these potentially competing approaches to public policy development and management practice are hard to untangle, as the distinction between policy and practice is itself highly blurred, as Ham (2009: 48) observed, 'it is clear that the implementation of policy feeds back into policymaking, making it difficult to draw hard and fast distinctions between these activities.'

Both the researcher and the practitioner can struggle to determine where their own beliefs and assumptions about policy and management perspectives, and the potential for a shared view on these, start and finish. This problem is bound to be particularly acute when the research in this area could be polarized into (a) narrative accounts of the development of policy and management which struggle to explain the causality in this complex environment, and (b) empirical studies which attempt to isolate cause and effect but concede this is difficult given the number of variables and multiple causes and consequences. Despite the problems, these perspectives begin to populate the canvas of the thesis topic. The further objective is to determine the precise nature of the research methodology. This approach could be either positive or normative. The research could adopt a quantitative or positivist approach, or it could adopt more qualitative or normative approach.

3.2 Selecting Methodologies to Appraise Healthcare Funding, Practitioner Views and Policy Development

Hospital funding, and funding for wider healthcare provider organisations, is complex and needs to be better understood if it is to be used to drive changes in the number and size of hospitals and their bed complements and change other types of healthcare facilities, via a market mechanism. These changes may well be necessary as the NHS attempts to move towards less hospital-based models of provision or may facilitate the provision of more efficient services overall. The first research question seeks to determine if structural factors drive particular hospitals' (and other NHS provider healthcare organisations') financial performance, which may be creating distortions in the market.

The academic underpinning of the market, based on New Public Management as described in Chapter 2, drives the need for a challenge to public producer interests, which could lead to market failure, which could drive enhanced efficiency. The first research question essentially seeks to establish if the existing funding arrangements, used up to the start of the pandemic could have delivered a market which can operate effectively, via testing practitioner views on the NHS funding approach. During the pandemic, in financial years 2020/21 and 2021/22 the normal NHS finance regime in England was suspended and replaced by a system that linked funding more closely to the costs of an organisation. Pre-pandemic the approach was more "fee for service", particularly for hospitals, and this is described later in this chapter.

The issue of how well this policy is implemented may be a function of how well the practitioners in the NHS market believe the system is and can operate. The second research question looks further at how appropriate practitioners in the NHS internal market believe the NHS internal market to be, and how deliverable it is, and these beliefs could be a large determinant of policy success. If good policy implementation at least in part depends upon 'street level bureaucrat' understanding and approval, what is thought by practitioners of NHS market policy is important but is perhaps little understood through formal research. If, therefore, in the context of the NHS internal market, NHS managers and finance practitioners have discretion as to how to interpret and implement the policy, and adopt it, this has a consequence for policy success that needs exploration.

The third research question then turns to how an individual or group of practitioners in the NHS internal market help to improve and advise on the system in place. There is a need to better understand the nature of policy formulation and the use of practitioner views and evidence in the development of policy. In this phase of the research, the author attempts to establish the views of key NHS stakeholders on the findings of this research, analysing their view on NHS market policy, and exploring the issues with them, along with the analysis from the first two thesis research questions. This seeks to understand different views on the English NHS market and to understand the role of policy and research evidence and how it drives the approach to policy. This element of the research reviews evidence and policy implementation literature, which is described in Chapter 5, alongside the results of the analysis of stakeholder views.

All three research questions have helped to enhance the author's understanding of the policy environment and how it is understood more generally. New ground for the author's understanding is around the policy implementation process and current alignment of views on the policy environment. Given that the NHS market once seemed to be here to stay (England has latterly perhaps caught up with Wales, Scotland or Northern Ireland, in abandoning elements of the internal market), it is worthwhile to see if practitioners think it could have ever operated effectively. During the twenty years from 1990 to 2010 in England, there seemed little formal appetite to fundamentally challenge the market's rationale and operation, although reports on healthcare integration from the Health Select Committee (2018) and the King's Fund (2010) started to make this case, and now the NHS Long Term Plan (2019) starts to make that case more overtly.

Fundamentally, the research seeks to examine the idea of good/bad policy and good/bad approaches to policy implementation. The research seeks to understand if practitioners believe the policy could work and is sensible or not, and then identify whether based on that conclusion they have been assisting fully in the implementation of the policy or not. The opportunity to bring the results of the first two phases of the research back to senior NHS figures to better understand their and indeed the author's views would seem to be a valuable line of inquiry.

3.3 Ethical Considerations and Access to Information and Participants

Some of the ethical concerns around access to policymakers and civil servants, the consequent impact of their views and their ability to speak freely and where there is a requirement for confidentially need addressing. Nobody within the NHS is cited in this work, although many colleagues have been involved in discussions with the author. Although there is a precise methodology for the three research questions within this thesis, the overall research has taken place through a wider framework of professional and managerial engagement. The precise approach to the three research questions could be best described by a notion of 'role-based emergent opportunism' – a term the author has coined. The author has essentially used his position in the NHS to access data and individuals to make the research possible. Without this insider status, the ability to interrogate and access the data used would be significantly harder, if not impossible, however, there are issues of power and insider status that are associated with this approach.

Figure 3.1 describes the chronology of the research and the author's changes in roles since 2008. In truth, the research process essentially stalled in 2012 due to an inability to easily access the required national datasets, whilst the author was working in Derby Hospitals. This was then made possible by the author's movement into a national role. This new role gave significantly greater access to a wide body of national data. This job move to a national role when also coupled with the author's nomination to serve on the HFMA Trustee body, gave invaluable access to both information and senior practitioners to canvass their views and opinions related to this area of study.

The ethical approval for the research design and approach was obtained within the School of Public Policy and Professional Practice at Keele at the time of the doctoral progression with the original doctoral supervisor. The research was considered low-risk and accorded with the policies and practices of Keele at the time of ethical review. The project was judged to be low-risk because the research was not contentious (e.g. animal research), it did not take place in a contentious context with vulnerable subjects (e.g. prison or school), did not involve procedures requiring pretence, based on research methods giving rise to consequences (e.g. causing personal distress). Furthermore, the project did not involve vulnerable subjects and did not involve the collection of personal data (Bottery and Wright (2019: 119).

Due to the organisational focus of this professional doctorate, various forms of consent were sought from the NHS and associated bodies: a) consent from the Directors of Finance for both NHSE and NHSI to use the data for RQ1, b) consent from the HFMA/PwC for the use of the data generated as part of the Marking Money Work in the health and care system (2018) for RQ2, and c) consent from the Chair of and the HFMA Policy and Research Committee and the HFMA CEO for the use of the HFMA Policy and Research Committee as a stakeholder group for RQ3. All the data, apart from that used for RQ1 was then anonymised. This organisational level data was already publicly available, in the main, although not in the format used for the analysis in the thesis.

The researcher took various precautions to ensure that the academic ethics system and those he worked with in professional practice were compatible. Throughout all the phases of the research, the author was open about the fact he was pursuing doctorate research at Keele University in NHS market policy and was keen to stress the benefits of participating in the research in practice and that being an important role for senior practitioners. The author has maintained the confidentiality of those who have been part of the research, apart from those cited in the acknowledgements. These processes followed the guidance set out by Cresswell (2009; 89).

The question of whether the internal market is, or could ever be, used as an approach to delivering healthcare efficiency, has been addressed by looking at data that the author managed to obtain whilst working in his national role. Although the data used are all publicly available, they have been obtained directly from the national NHS management tier, meaning that the data have been compiled from national sources, which saved a huge amount of time, by getting the data in a format that was aggregated for all NHS provider organisations, in a common way. Such analysis of this secondary data is, the author believes, the first time that the overall English NHS's financial performance has ever been analysed so comprehensively, by a relatively independent practitioner-researcher, to try and understand and influence policy.

Figure 3.1 - Research Chronology and the Author's Changes in Roles

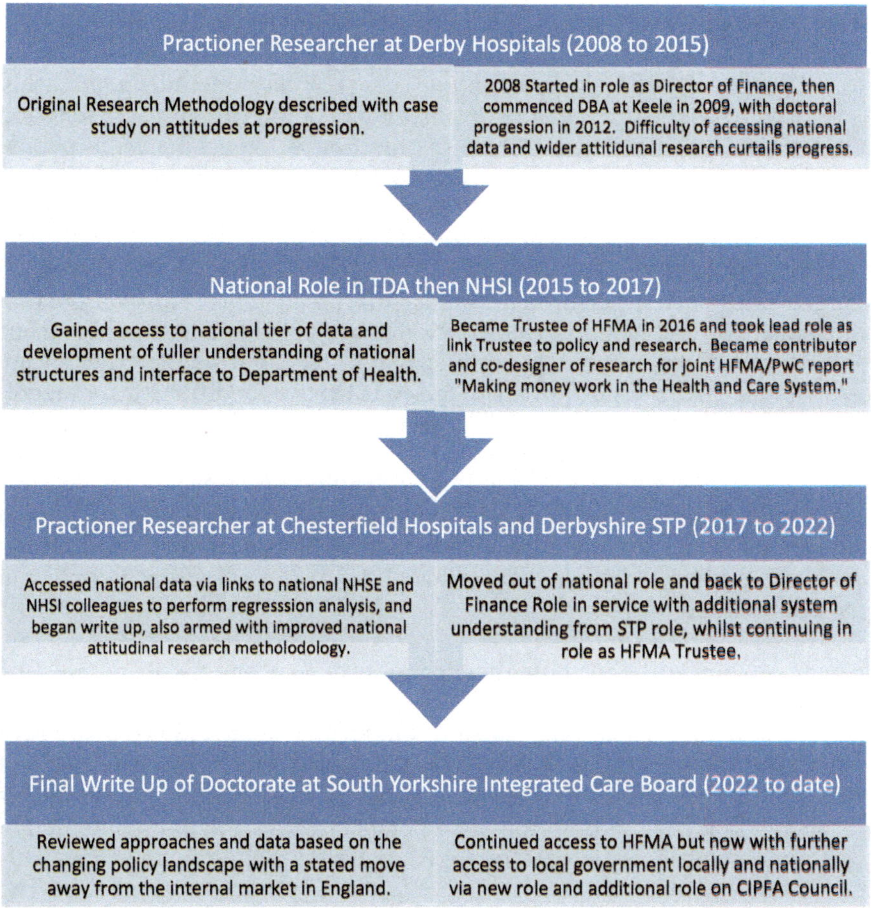

Practitioner Researcher at Derby Hospitals (2008 to 2015)

Original Research Methodology described with case study on attitudes at progression.

2008 Started in role as Director of Finance, then commenced DBA at Keele in 2009, with doctoral progession in 2012. Difficulty of accessing national data and wider attitidunal research curtails progress.

National Role in TDA then NHSI (2015 to 2017)

Gained access to national tier of data and development of fuller understanding of national structures and interface to Department of Health.

Became Trustee of HFMA in 2016 and took lead role as link Trustee to policy and research. Became contributor and co-designer of research for joint HFMA/PwC report "Making money work in the Health and Care System."

Practitioner Researcher at Chesterfield Hospitals and Derbyshire STP (2017 to 2022)

Accessed national data via links to national NHSE and NHSI colleagues to perform regresssion analysis, and began write up, also armed with improved national attitudinal research metholodology.

Moved out of national role and back to Director of Finance Role in service with additional system understanding from STP role, whilst continuing in role as HFMA Trustee.

Final Write Up of Doctorate at South Yorkshire Integrated Care Board (2022 to date)

Reviewed approaches and data based on the changing policy landscape with a stated move away from the internal market in England.

Continued access to HFMA but now with further access to local government locally and nationally via new role and additional role on CIPFA Council.

The author's changing role during the time of the research, is perhaps of particular interest. At the professional doctorate inception stage, the author - although an insider - could perhaps openly criticize the nature of policy since the Derby role had no influence over policy. Although the author's next role provided access to the data, he was then more associated with policy determination, which would have made overtly critical conclusions associated with the policy approach potentially problematic. Now having developed the national linkages and access to the resources required to access the data, he has returned to a role which makes a critique of national policy easier. There is a further paradox here in the role of the practitioner-researcher: at the stage of his career where the author was potentially more able to influence a change in national NHS finance policy, he felt less able to make that change in terms of agency and ability to challenge the dominant ideology. Drake and Heath (2011: 19) noted:

> People at work in...institutions of all kinds operate in intensely political climates. Dominant ideologies allow for little dissent and create practices through the distribution of power between people in the organisation and through dominant sets of relations regarding practice. It is quite impossible for people operating in these regimes to ignore the dominant practices.

The regression analysis performed and then discussed helps to answer the first research question and looks for a correlation between the financial performance of NHS organisations and other factors which could be contributing to healthcare organisation's financial performance, to see if the preconditions for a market may have existed, which is then discussed with other finance practitioners. This section of the research (presented in Chapter 4) will help to describe the complexity of English NHS funding, given the different funding streams and approaches in place. It sought through discussions with practitioners to evaluate their understanding and views on the robustness of these funding mechanisms and see whether they believed the funding approach could run an internal market.

There are several different potential research design options to answer the second research question. Firstly, the nature of a question around the attitudes of the practitioners in a particular system could lend itself to either a qualitative or quantitative approach. Secondly, the author could write a narrative account examining his own views on the system and potentially fully describe his own epistemological and/or ontological perspective, based on the interaction between his practitioner perspective lived experience and the newer insights gained from the doctoral study process, via a reflective approach. The generation of this knowledge would have benefits to the author, but may not reveal much about the wider perspective of other practitioners on the NHS internal market. These two approaches to the research do begin to reveal a particular challenge for social science research about the nature of knowledge and how the interplay between a social construction of reality and an actual 'empirical' reality that may occur or exist.

In terms of the author's research therefore it is worth noting this duality in terms of observing the development of NHS quasi-market policies. Perhaps, the subjective statement "markets are good and drive efficiency" has become an objective fact. Perhaps the statement "Payments by Results has been a key policy instrument in driving the improvements we have seen in the

English NHS over recent years" has also become a fact. In essence, the second research question seeks to ascertain what current practitioner views are on such issues. By its very nature, however, the proposed approach to research cannot evaluate the extent to which practitioners' answers to such questions are being generated by the cumulative impact of cultural capital accumulation and/or power references or structures, which will have contributed to and created such views within practitioners.

Noting the tensions between objective and subjective knowledge, there is now a need to move precisely onto the second research question related to practitioner views. There are a few ways that data can be collected which can begin to describe the views or attitudes of a particular group of research participants in a particular field of study. A questionnaire can be developed and used to generate qualitative or quantitative data. A survey or interview can be used which can then be coded with its responses to create quantitative data. It is also possible to undertake several structured, semi-structured or unstructured interviews, several focus groups could be performed which generate qualitative data on the subject area.

The author piloted a questionnaire-based approach to generate quantitative data on practitioners' views on the NHS market reforms as part of his pre-progression doctoral work. If this were useful in the final study it would be tending towards a more closed, and perhaps objectivist, research approach. This pre-Progression work developed an approach to collating attitudes to the NHS market in a pilot study. This work sought to ascertain the level of understanding and belief on levels of adoption and practitioner approval of NHS market policy. Through the research period the approach to collecting attitudinal research, on the internal market changed, due to an opportunity afforded to the author, related to his role in the Policy and Research Committee for HFMA. This role allowed him to access a wider range of qualitative practitioner opinions on NHS finance and the NHS internal market regime, through joint work between HFMA and PwC, in 2015.

Through the emergence of the HFMA/PwC work the author gained access to an approach to generate objective and subjective data. He was able to influence this new approach to data collection by being part of the stakeholder group designing and commissioning the project. Here both approaches were included via both closed and open questions, to many practitioners, which were then followed up by the action research phase of the thesis. The precise approach to the attitudinal research is presented in Chapter 5 where the author's contribution to a HFMA/PwC Report is described, in addition to the findings. The overall research approach is represented in Figure 3.2.

Originally for the third phase of the research, the author had intended to interview a number of key stakeholders in NHS finance and discuss with them the results of the first two stages of the research, (a) associated with the adequacy of funding system to technically deliver an internal market for health, and (b) the extent to which practitioners in the NHS finance field ever believe this was an adequate approach and helped to either support or usurp the policy. The approach taken to seek stakeholders' views on their ability to shape and influence NHS Finance policy will be described in Chapter 6 and utilises the author's role as a Trustee and active participant in the HFMA Policy and Research Committee and uses this forum via an action research methodology.

Figure 3.2 - The interrelationship between the three central research approaches

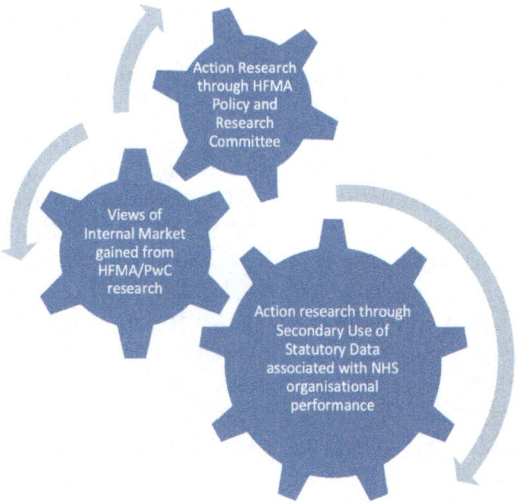

3.4 Abductive, Action and Practitioner Research and Ongoing Enquiry

The research attempts to address issues concerning the effectiveness and potential desirability of the internal market. Given the nature of the data in this area, it is suggested that the absolute assessment of the effectiveness and desirability of the policy and its development will also require the collection and interpretation of a range of qualitative as well as quantitative data. This qualitative data will look at finance practitioners' views on the advantages and disadvantages of the quasi-market system. The third element of the research, in Chapter 6, will also be more reflexive and will look at how the first two elements of the research are informing the author's view of the quasi-market policy environment, and all have an action research strand as the work is disseminated and discussed with practitioners in the field of NHS management and finance.

The claimed positivist perspective for the research can be challenged in terms of the ability to reach such conclusions. Cresswell's (2009: 6) definition of 'worldview' was important in shaping the methodology.

> **worldview** as meaning "a basic set of beliefs that guide action" (Guba, 1990, p.17). Others have called them paradigms (Lincoln and Guba, 2000; Mertens, 1998); epistemologies and ontologies (Crotty, 1998), or broadly conceived research methodologies (Neuman, 2000)." He "sees worldviews as a general orientation about the world and the nature of research that a researcher holds.

The four worldviews Cresswell identifies are (i) post-positivism (determination, reductionism, empirical observation and measurement, and theory verification), (ii) social constructivism (understanding, multiple participant meanings, social and historical construction and theory generation), (iii) Advocacy/participatory (political, empowered issue-orientated, collaborative and change-orientated), and (iv) Pragmatism (consequences of actions, problem centred, pluralistic and real-world practice orientated). On reading these definitions and types of potential enquiry it is unsurprising perhaps that a mixed methods approach was selected for the research. Essentially, the author wishes to draw some firm conclusions about the nature of the NHS quasi-market but would acknowledge the difficulty of observing the social phenomenon in this way, perhaps from a post-positivist perspective. There is also an acknowledgement that as a practitioner in this field there is a bias associated with this perspective and that individuals develop subjective meanings of their experiences and perspectives: a social constructivist perspective (Blaikie (2007)).

The author further notes that the system under examination is a highly politicised one and that social policy concerning quasi-market development has a particular political dimension in terms of thoughts around the efficacy or otherwise of the prevailing economic system and markets. This social policy and marketisation may be marginalising groups or individuals in society, this is known as an Advocacy/Participatory perspective. And above all other aims of the research, the author would wish to draw conclusions which could practically identify a research approach which engages with the problems of the existing system to seek opportunities for real-world practice improvement, a pragmatic perspective. In short, therefore, the research aims have the potential to be wide and require marshalling to ensure that the scope of the research is both practically deliverable, and has a well-defined theoretical perspective, despite the potential plural nature of the theoretical perspective(s) that are associated with the approach.

The development of the NHS internal market continues to be a highly discussed area of public policy debate. The previous Health Bill (2011), which resulted in the 2012 Act, built on the previous stages of quasi-market development has several current and ongoing challenges identified by NHS Confederation (2011): (a) complexity of commissioning structures, (b) consequent difficulties in decision making, (c) over-centralisation and slow delegation of power, (d) accountability, (e) enabling competition and integration, (f) quality of care and (g) how failing organisations will be managed. All these issues were pertinent to the research and continue despite the 2022 Act.

The nature of knowledge around research tends to fall into four broad arenas, in the opinion of the author. First, there is practitioner understanding and participation in the systems and their development. Given the 'role-based emergent opportunism' research approach of the author and the fact that he has a full-time role as a Director of Finance in the system, this practitioner approach is dominant in influencing the research and the understanding of knowledge in the area. Second, there is then a wide strand of contemporary commentary on the development of the system and its consequential impact which is not particularly influenced by a theoretical perspective. The Health Service Journal (the managerial trade press for NHS management), for example, covers issues such as the development of the NHS market and the potential tensions between competition and integration of services. There is also commentary from organisations like the King's Fund and Nuffield Trust which are UK charities set up to improve the formulation of health policy. A study was also published by the Office of Health Economics (2012) on "Competition in the NHS", which added a framework for discussing competition and its role in the NHS, which added to the body of knowledge. Neither of these first two arenas often has a stated or cited theoretical perspective.

Third, there are then a wide number of academic practitioners, such as Le Grand, Pollock and Paton who have actively researched and commentated on the NHS and its marketisation. Their research and for the others operating in the field can vary very widely, (to force perhaps arbitrarily into the worldviews of Cresswell) from the Post-Positive approach of Cooper, Gibbons, Jones and McGuire, to the Social Constructivism of Paton, or the Advocacy/Participatory approach of Pollock, or the Pragmatism of Le Grand. The fourth area of knowledge is relatively underdeveloped in the author's opinion and that is the role of practitioner-based research into social policy and management practice development in the NHS and perhaps more widely. On this fourth area, it is interesting that many senior medical practitioners continue to see their role as researchers, which appears to be less prevalent, in the author's experience, for senior NHS managers and senior finance practitioners.

A key tension in the proposed research is that of objectivity, bias or power which can subvert the research, which is conducted by a practitioner. Despite there being an obvious benefit of practitioner-based research, predominantly the knowledge accumulated by the researcher in their area of expertise, this can lead to an inability to remain objective due to how their practice creates a social construct in which the practitioner operates. The duality of the role between active participants in the subject area, and researchers (who can claim to maintain a certain distance from the issues in question) has been hard to deliver.

There are then further ethical issues associated with the practitioner being an 'insider' in their chosen field. A pragmatic approach to these issues would allow such tensions to be clearly stated, where it was possible to identify them, without getting so side-lined by reductionist enquiry that it prevents some conclusions being drawn, and then trying to provide advice around improving the approach to an important area of public policy. Drake and Heath (2011: 29) noted:

> There are clear sets of difficulties in conducting a research study in one's own workplace in terms of the researcher's status within the institution and considerations regarding what the researcher represents to the other participants. Drake (2009) suggests that with this style of working comes privileged access to participants, although this comes with a health warning since the researcher must live with the consequences of their project, and ethical dimensions need careful consideration.

In the context of this research, the 'institution' in which the author is intending to research is the whole of the English NHS, as opposed to being the organisation which holds the researcher's contract of employment – 'NHS South Yorkshire – Integrated Care Board'. There could be significant ethical considerations associated with the author having access to data and information on his own organisation if a single organisation case study approach were adopted. There is perhaps less concern if the research is conducted away from the employing organisation. However, the NHS has a relatively small senior finance and management community and firm conclusions which potentially identify significant frailties in the existing system, were they to become apparent, would need relatively careful and skilful handling to protect the research subjects and potentially the author. From this perspective, the 'institution' being studied would be the English NHS, and although the author tends to regard his contract of employment as being with the NHS, as opposed to the subset of the NHS which happens to be signatory to his contract of employment, protecting the author and research participants is important. This research being wider than his own employing organisation removes some of the tension identified by Drake and Heath. There are concerns around the practitioner and the conclusions regarding the policy environment across the English NHS, the impact of the author's standing within that environment and the impact of the research findings on it, which will need to be evaluated and described through the proposed action research phase of the thesis particularly.

Despite the tensions around research perspectives and approaches, which do require acknowledgement and consideration, Scanlon (2000: 2) notes that:

> ...research is carried out to fulfil one or more of the following objectives:
>
> - To contribute to a particular discipline (for example, psychology).
> - To inform policy (for example, policy on housing, crime, education).
> - To address a specific issue or problem (for example, drug taking in a local school).

The research herein attempts to address all three of these objectives. The research hopefully contributes to the academic public policy and management and economics fields through the analysis by addressing issues regarding the effectiveness of quasi-market structures. In Chapter 2, positive and narrative accounts of the effectiveness of NHS market structures have been identified. This research has attempted both a positivist and a narrative account approach. During the third element of the research, the author particularly wanted to be able to address the findings of the first two elements of research to other members of the NHS's financial management community, via action research. Bowling (2009: 441) described:

> Action research is undertaken by participants in social situations to improve their practices and their understanding of them. The method was designed to study social systems with the aim of changing them (i.e., to achieve certain goals).

The selection of research design tries to be mindful of the different practitioner views on the development of the quasi-market, whilst trying to influence professional practice through a pragmatic, mixed methods approach. The initial part of the research design attempts to test some of the underlying beliefs of practitioners around what factors could be causing 'good' and 'bad' financial results in the English NHS to see if they believe a market mechanism is possible with the post-1989 and current NHS funding arrangements. These financial results are important if hospital success and ongoing financial standing are dependent upon them. The author would further assert that financial reporting and funding in the English NHS is so complicated that this analysis would best be delivered by someone actively working in this field. To derive a worthwhile set of conclusions in this area requires a close working knowledge of how the system operates given its complexity.

3.5 Is NHS Funding Sophisticated Enough to Run a Market?

The first research question, therefore, attempts to identify how effectively the NHS internal market is operating. For there to be an effective internal market mechanism which benefits from the efficiency produced by a market (if we subscribe to a particular micro and macro-economic 'worldview') there needs to be an effective series of pricing and other market structures to create an effective market approach. The English NHS is funded by a national tariff for many hospital services, which attempts to ensure each hospital gets the same payment for the same treatment and care. The first research question that the thesis poses is "Do finance practitioners believe the way in which the NHS is funded could run a market?". Essentially here the author's practitioner knowledge of NHS funding structures was required to address this research aim. The author wished to examine the potential frailty or robustness of the internal market by looking at any correlation between healthcare organisations' financial performance (surplus/deficit) and several independent variables. Often the debate about hospital and healthcare competition tends to be hijacked, in the author's view, by the issue of the potential entrance to the market of the private sector. There is also a need to better understand how the existing funding approach is fairly reimbursing existing NHS providers. The variables included in the first element of the research, including all English NHS providers, use a bivariate regression analysis between financial performance and potential causal factors for that financial performance. The independent variables and the hypothesis that were tested are described below:

1. **Organisational Turnover** – Is it easier or harder for smaller or larger NHS provider organisations to make surpluses? Therefore, should some infrastructure funding arrive as a separate funding stream to hospitals if they are to continue in their existing configuration, to enable a market to work?
2. **Reference Cost Index** – This is a national measure of comparative unit cost efficiency and should identify the organisation's opportunity for surplus generation by denoting comparative efficiency. If the measure does not denote comparative efficiency,

it may need to be amended and improved. If a market is to work, organisations with lower costs should be better able to make surpluses.

3. **Reference Cost Quantum as a Proportion of Turnover** – This is a measure of the alternative sources of income a Trust receives beyond the direct patient care income, it could be a measure of diversification of the Trust, with potential approaches to that diversification being more education and training, research, charitable or other non-core NHS service funding. It seeks to explore how core NHS funding may be sufficient to run an NHS organisation.

4. **CCG to Provider interdependence** – Does the proportion of the main CCGs spend with their local hospital or healthcare provider determine financial health, either positively or negatively? In areas of the health system where there is a closer engagement between provider and commissioner, could this lead to collusive behaviour or a more mature whole health economy approach?

5. **CCG Surplus/Deficit** – Is the provider surplus or deficit-neutral to the local commissioner's financial performance, and therefore what does this mean about the potential distribution of financial risk in the system, and consequently the maturity of the market approach?

6. **CCG Funding Position against Target** – Some CCGs are closer or further from the financial allocation which a national funding formula suggests they should receive. Does this impact their local Trust provider's financial health, and whether or not this is creating a market distortion?

7. **Market Forces Factor (MFF)** – All Trusts have a different assumed rate of cost due to geographical location, (MFF), but perhaps a more structured review of how the NHS pays each hospital and funds each CCG differentially according to their geographic location needs to be undertaken, to see if a distortion is created?

8. The proportion of **Income generated from Nationally Commissioned Services** versus locally commissioned services from the CCGs - The scope of services offered by NHS organisations are all different as they provide a different proportion of services covered by services which are commissioned from CCGs as opposed to services that are commissioned nationally. It could be that national or locally commissioned service proportions may be a driver of financial performance.

9. The impact of the **Private Finance Initiative (PFI)** – Some NHS finance practitioners and wider commentators have asserted that

PFI has created a poor competitive advantage for those hospitals which have rebuilt hospitals using this funding approach. There is a debate therefore on the transparency of the funding for PFI hospitals now needed and the extent to which this creates a market distortion.

10. Hospital **Research and Education Income** – A separate funding stream exists for Trusts which undertake non-commercial research and the education of doctors and nurses. This income is removed from the reference cost quantum prior to calculation. This is a slightly narrower indicator than that used in variable 3, above. In terms of how the Reference Costing System works, if the research and education income is not in line with cost, then the subsequent healthcare costs will be inaccurate.

11. **CQC Rating** – Following discussion at the HFMA Policy and Research Committee, the group were particularly keen to see the extent to which English healthcare organisations' CQC rating was correlated to the organisation's financial performance. Is higher or lower quality, measured by CQC rating, correlated with better or worse financial performance?

12. **Emergency Department (ED) Four-Hour Wait Performance** – Also, the same discussion at the HFMA Policy and Research Committee sought to see whether improved financial performance was costing the organisation in terms of the delivery of the key target associated with hospital performance, the Four-Hour waiting for standard in the Emergency Department. Is higher or lower performance target delivery correlated with better or worse financial performance?

The data for many of these variables are publicly available but the author used his insider status to gain some of the required information from NHS England (the lead Commissioning authority in the English NHS) and NHS Improvement (his previous employer and the former Provider regulator for NHS provider bodies). One of the benefits of the practitioner's status is that he has ready access to both these organisations – NHSE and NHSI – and the Department of Health. He has shared his research approach with senior colleagues at all three of these organisations and there has been significant support for these lines of enquiry. He also tested the variables selected, via a review of those variables and the potential for the use of others within the regression analysis, via the HFMAs Policy and Research Committee.

3.6 What are Finance Practitioners' Attitudes, and have they Impacted on Policy Success?

The second research question that the thesis poses is **"Have the views of finance practitioners on the internal market impacted policy success and policy persistence?"**. Attitudinal research is a user-experience research method which is used to understand a respondent's opinions, beliefs, feelings or thoughts. For this thesis, this information was gathered via 203 questionnaire responses in 2017, and through further and ongoing supporting conversations with NHS finance practitioners. A questionnaire approach was piloted with practitioners in NHS finance and medical roles as part of the preliminary work for the doctorate. As the purpose of this research question is to establish what practitioners think - and believe - about the NHS internal market system there are difficulties relating to forming concrete conclusions from the approach. This attitudinal research reveals two different types of issues, considerations, and perhaps problems, with the English NHS system: a) it reveals flaws (perceived and real problems) with the system(s), and b) it reveals how the system impacts on the motivation and beliefs of NHS managers and staff.

This second area of research needed to be mindful of the interaction between the researcher and research participants, in terms of ethical considerations. It also had the potential, to reveal some interesting tensions between those developing public policy and those living with, and through, the implementation of such policies. Irrespective of the approach to gathering data (questionnaires, interviews, organisational ethnographies, focus groups) on practitioner perspectives and attitudes on the NHS market approach there are ethical issues for the qualitative research phase as noted by Silverman (2011: 428):

> According to the professional guidelines, the researcher is responsible for the informed consent, for trust and protection, and for protecting the participants' privacy by confidentiality. A signed consent form then becomes a guarantee that participants are informed about the research and consent to participate.

Despite the real ethical concerns, the author wishes to develop a further ongoing relationship with his colleagues, to try and understand the wider collective effort needed to potentially improve the system in which practitioners operate. This will hopefully mean an ongoing dialogue and acknowledgement that in this field there is not a static research problem. The methodology selected for the attitudinal research aims to encourage a relatively open dialogue with the researcher, that will enable a sharing of ideas and best practice and views which will seek to build upon existing knowledge in the research area. Initially, the use of the HFMA blog and then the availability of the Policy and Research

Committee of the HFMA provides a research feedback forum for the thesis, and a vehicle for the approach to dissemination of the findings.

The proposed approach to the second research question involved gathering data on attitudes to NHS market structures. The research design needed to ensure that the research objectives of this phase of the thesis were clear. The nature of the data generated from a relatively simple questionnaire needed to ensure that specific research questions are posed as described by Bryman and Burgess (1994: 174):

> In applied policy research, qualitative methods are used to meet a variety of different objectives. The questions that need to be addressed will vary from study to study but broadly they can be divided into four categories; contextual: identifying the nature and form of what exists; diagnostic – examining the reasons for, or causes of, what exists; evaluative – appraising the effectiveness of what exists; and, strategic – identifying new theories, policies, plans or actions.

The purpose of the questionnaire phase of the research was to evaluate the contextual issues around attitudes and perceptions that are held. Through the research design, it was thought appropriate to link the questionnaires and the ongoing action orientation of the research into some semi-structured interviews and focus groups to tease out practitioner understanding of what generated these attitudes and to gain alternate perspectives on how the systems could be improved. The attitudinal research phase will seek to address three key areas of practitioner understanding of the quasi-market, (i) their level of understanding of the policy environment, (ii) the level of implementation of the policy as they perceive its impact in their organisations, and (iii) their support or otherwise for the policy and whether they believe it is having a favourable impact on healthcare delivery in England.

The purpose of this element of the research was to determine the extent to which an attitudinal questionnaire on quasi-market reform could adequately capture practitioner views. It began to reveal what those views were, and because of the pilot study, the author began to develop a better understanding of his views on policies. The developing view of the author began to solidify the approach to the second research question. It was originally proposed that this research question was solely addressed via a questionnaire. This approach was piloted to examine whether the approach was likely to adequately answer the research question or to see whether an alternative approach to the data collection was required. A pilot study reviewed the appropriateness of both the questionnaire-based research approach, questionnaire design and other issues associated with research; and what the author could do differently around the final research design, based upon the pilot study findings.

In common with much practitioner-based research at the doctoral level in the social sciences, the research strategy eventually chosen was an Abductive Research Strategy, as described by Burgess, Sieminski and Arthur (2006). As the study is largely addressing attitudes, there is a need to understand the context of those attitudes and inner and outer meanings. This approach is further described by Blaikie (2007: 107):

- Abduction, a strategy that is implicit in several research paradigms, has been advocated as either the only suitable one for the social sciences or as an essential adjunct to other research strategies.
- Abduction characterizes those research paradigms concerned with deriving expert accounts of social life from the everyday accounts that social actors can provide.
- Since much of social life is routine and habitual, and takes place in an unreflective, taken-for-granted manner, the accounts of social actors do not usually reveal the largely tacit meanings that underpin their interactions.

Abduction, the process of re-visiting material but retaining the authenticity of the voices that it contains (as has taken place with the coding of the interviews), is explained below:

> The main access a researcher has to these constructions is through the knowledge that social actors use in the production, reproduction, and interpretation of the phenomenon under investigation. Their reality, the way they have constructed and interpreted their activities together, is embedded in their everyday language. Hence, the researcher has to enter their world in order to discover the motives and reasons that accompany social activities. (Blaikie, 2007: 10)

The perspectives of the practitioners in the NHS and NHS finance are probably both explicitly and implicitly understood. It is therefore difficult to be able to separate both the inner perspectives of the Practitioner, from a more objective view of the overall policy environment and reality. Figure 3.1, from Bruyn, explores this dichotomy and tension and tries to tease out the tension between subjective and objective knowledge. Although the initial intention of the research was to try and occupy the "traditional empiricist" perspective there was a gradual realisation through the course of the research period that the author increasingly realised that he was occupying (and could only occupy) the perspective of a "participant observer".

Table 3.1 - The Human Perspective: Methodological Dimensions - Bruyn (1963)

	Inner Perspective (Participant Observer)	**Outer Perspective** (Traditional Empiricist)
Philosophical foundation	Idealism	Naturalism
Mode of: Interpretation	Concrete procedures	Operational procedures
Conceptualization	Sensitizing concepts	Formal concepts
Description	Synthesis	Analysis
Explanation: Principles	Telic	Causal
Models	Voluntarism	Deterministic
Aims	Sensitively accurate Interpretation and explanation of man's social and cultural life	Accurate measurement and prediction of man's behaviour

Researchers using an abductive research strategy often undertake observation and live and breathe their research. Participant observation can take many forms, and this doctoral research process (with the researcher having worked inside these environments) embodies this process, and the process is concerned with the Inner Perspectives identified.

It was felt that the finance practitioners' views themselves needed to be heard in this research process. So, the HFMA/PwC report, and the responses to the survey used to generate it, were further analysed for this study, with over 200 participants; then the Policy and Research Committee conversations; followed by rigorous reduction, whilst maintaining the authenticity of the interviewees' responses (Kvale and Brinkmann, 2009) was thought essential, and in keeping with the wider research aims.

This moved away from the original proposal associated with the piloted questionnaire on practitioner views. This new approach enabled the researcher to:

Re-describe these actions and motives, and the situations in which they occur, in the technical language of social scientific discourse. Individual motives and actions have to be abstracted into typical motives for typical situations. These social scientific typifications provide an understanding of the activities and may then become ingredients in more systematic explanatory accounts. (Blaikie, 2007: 10).

Bhaskar (1978) describes the abductive strategy in terms of layers, where the members of the group under scrutiny have their insider understanding scrutinized by the researcher and made available for the wider 'outside' world. Blaikie also explains this in terms of layers. The columns in Figure 3.2 demonstrate the adaptation of the Bhaskar original, as identified by Blaikie. This has the explanation of the generic abductive attitudinal research strategy explained in the first column of the table, alongside this doctoral research process with specific examples from this thesis, in the second column of the table.

One of the basic differences in research strategies is whether a researcher is choosing to use a top-down or bottom-up approach. This revised attitudinal research process was conducted inside the NHS on the NHS internal market itself, to find out what respondents, including the author, in the NHS thought. Hence, a bottom-up approach was adopted, as the participants' voices being heard was an important part of this process. This is important as the effectiveness of policy, may not just be determined by the coherence of the policy itself, but also by the acceptance of the policy from the practitioners within the area which the policy is trying to influence. If a top-down approach had been taken, using quantitative approaches to data, such as the piloted attitudinal questionnaire: perhaps asking what and when questions, rather than open-ended questions a different standpoint would have been adopted.

The ongoing Policy and Research conversations encouraged practitioners to explain their positioning via their accounts. A top-down approach would have resulted in a very different form of practise-based enquiry, where statistics could have been generated on the numbers of those who saw the NHS in a particular way (Cohen et al, 2007), rather than the question that was asked on the reasons as to why the NHS was functioning as it currently does or does not. What has been learnt from the internal markets adoption process, is of importance, for this element of the research - for these results directly from the qualitative motivations of senior staff: who change such a system, when change is complex and ambiguous.

Table 3.2 - Attitudinal Research Strategy: Adapted from Bhaskar by Blaikie (2007)

Everyday concepts and meanings	Statement: There is and has been an internal market in health
Provide the basis for	
Social action/interaction	Choice: Is this working, or creating a worse bureaucracy or unintended consequences
About which	
Social actors can give accounts	Finance Practitioners and wider perspectives on the English NHS
From which	
Social scientific description can be made	In vivo coding of these accounts provides the opportunity to give the detail of the micro positioning of leaders in the system, then further discussed with social actors, via HFMA Policy and Research Committee
From which	
Social theories can be generated	A macro social scientific position can be generated relating to the functioning and appropriateness of the internal market
Or which can be understood in terms of existing	
Social theories or perspectives	Theories and perspectives on markets, public service and targets.

Therefore, since the more "traditional empirical" pilot study was conducted the author has been considering the best approach to getting a good overall sample of practitioner views on NHS Finance and the internal market, to better understand their social construction and perspective on policy. The author finally settled on using NHS finance practitioners, as he became increasingly interested in them specifically as an epistemic community, as opposed to a broader pilot research sample. Although the findings of the pilot study did have some highly interesting results on different professional views on the internal market, the specific finance epistemic community was chosen, as the author recognised the importance and meaning of these "participant observers".

Before reviewing the approach to abductive research, the author intended to explore the use of a web-based tool such as SurveyMonkey to help generate responses to a series of questions trialled as a pilot study. The author also considered targeting a medical, surgical, finance and Chief Executive cohort for his research questions. These four groupings of practitioners could reveal interesting differences in attitudes by introducing two additional, or even further types of practitioners. Also, the author considered looking at the alignment of a hospital executive team around their attitudes to the English NHS market, to potentially see what this could mean about team alignment and potential organisational performance. The first research aim sought to review the nature of hospital financial performance and the variables that cause this. A further variable could potentially be the "Common and aligned Executive Team view" on NHS market structures, which could be an indicator of good and consistent organisational leadership. Eventually, though the final methodology selected sought to look specifically at NHS finance practitioner views and understand their specific "participant observer" perspectives on the internal market, as a grouping which the author specifically represented via his HFMA and CIPFA roles.

In terms of the 'role-based emergent opportunism' approach to the research, therefore, the author, due to his role within the HFMA as a Trustee, was keen to localise the research with the NHS finance "Community of Practice" (Wenger, 1998). When, therefore the author was presented with an opportunity to work with HFMA and PwC on a project looking at how NHS finance needed some element of renewal, which (as part of it) was going to build from a previous PwC report which had made recommendations on changing the NHS system architecture, he thought this would be a useful vehicle to give his research better reach and potential impact. Although the author was also aware of the bias that may be prevalent in jointly undertaking the work with PwC and HFMA, and the fact that participants in the research, and respondents to the report, may view it in a particular way, (due to the nature of both organisations), this was believed to be likely to have a better dissemination impact. It resulted in a specific report which sought to influence practice and gave rise to a broader range of data and legitimacy within his epistemic group than if the author had pursued the research independently.

The data from the finance survey approach is discussed in Chapter 5. In addition to taking the verbatim responses the survey, this thesis research also used coding on these responses to identify key issues/themes and views from practitioners. The author has used NVivo (and for the rest of his coding analysis from the survey) to code the 93 responses. The details as to why the respondents had these views have been coded in different themes, but the responses did not easily lend themselves to auto-coding. Coding is described by Cresswell (2009: 186):

> Coding is the process of organising the material into chunks or segments of text before bringing meaning to information ...It involves taking text data or pictures gathered during the data collection, segmenting sentences (or paragraphs) or images into categories, and labelling these categories with a term based on the actual language of the participant (called an in vivo term).

The coding of all the qualitative data was time-consuming and involved the eight steps process further elaborated upon by Cresswell, namely, (i) getting a sense of all the responses, (ii) dissecting the thoughts of some of the more interesting responses initially, (iii) once completed for several respondents make a list of topics/codes, (iv) go back to the data with this coded list to see if new topics emerge, (v) find the most descriptive wording for the topics, (vi) make a final decision on the codes, (vii) assemble all the data belonging to each category (in this case each question response), then (viii) code the data.

The author then had an opportunity to discuss this report and his subsequent coding analysis of the data further developed from the survey, with twenty colleagues in the HFMA Policy and Research Committee. Whilst delivering the first two research questions, the research will also seek to address issues of public policy implementation and examine the understanding of participants on the theoretical underpinning of the NHS internal market, via the conversations derived from the HFMA/PwC research questionnaire. The research tries to create a bridge between theory and practice, which is important for the third research question.

3.7 Are Finance Practitioners an Epistemic Community Able to Influence Policy?

The third research question that the thesis poses is "*To what extent do finance practitioners inside the NHS constitute an epistemic community which is able to influence the development of policy and advocate a move away from the internal market?*". This action research aim was broad and attempted to examine the space between public policy and policy implementation. The approach and ambition for the action research phase, described below by Stringer (2007) was therefore to try and facilitate a debate and reach conclusions, with finance practitioners, on how to improve the English NHS system.

> Formally, then, action research, in its most effective forms, is phenomenological (focusing on people's actual lived experience/ reality), interpretive (focusing on their interpretation of acts and activities), and hermeneutic (incorporating the meaning people make of events in their lives). It provides the means by which stakeholders – those centrally investigated by the issue investigated – explore their experience, gain greater clarity and understanding of the events and activities, and use those extended understandings to construct effective solutions to problem(s) on which the study was focused. (Stringer (2007); 20)

The purpose of the research was, therefore, to allow a reflexive approach by the author, with some of his NHS colleagues, to explore the policy approaches to NHS management and financial management and propose potential improvements to those approaches. Based on the Stringer definition the research aimed to: favourably impact upon the understanding of practitioners, around the impact and understanding of the policy environment; further, to understand how they interpret the policy environment; and, how practitioners perceive what is shaping their understanding of the environment in which they operate. At a less ambitious, but more deliverable level, it was also hoped that the research itself would enable the author to better understand, and deal with, the tensions associated with the applied policy framework which should make his working life (and potentially his colleagues' lives) slightly easier to understand, explain, rationalise, and only possibly change.

3.8 Research and Career Overlaps: Biases and Opportunities

The three phases of the research summarised, therefore, are:

1. Quantitative regression analysis sought to identify the correlations

between good and bad financial performance in English NHS provider organisations with selected independent variables. It was based on available secondary data, (which the author had access to in his professional capacity) and is then discussed with the HFMA Policy and Research Committee. This data described in Chapter 4. The data was made available to the author by the Directors of Finance of NHSE and NHSI. The author had to manipulate and analyse this data in Excel and then discussed this analysis with the HFMA Policy and Research Committee.

2. Attitudinal research which reviewed understanding, the scale of impact and the level of support for quasi-market policies with the English NHS, was pursued via the HFMA/PwC joint work. This data was made available to the author via the approval of the rest of the Steering Group associated with the report, which the author was a member of. The author had to code this data which is described in Chapter 5.

3. An action research phase which sought to provide the results of the first two research objectives, back to practitioners, operating within the NHS quasi-market area: extending both their and the author's understanding of these policies and their impacts, through the HFMA Policy and Research Committee, which is described in Chapter 6 and Appendices 7 to 17.

Figure 3.3 gives further context to the role of the author, the changing nature of the research design and how that has been impacted by the evolution of the English NHS internal market and calls for and moves away from it. It outlines how the author's approach to the research – specifically related to RQ1 – turned away from an empirical approach to funding to a focus on practitioner views on the funding approach. It notes the development of the thinking towards practitioner policy adoption roles and policy influence and the role of the NHS finance epistemic committee informing the approach to RQ2 and RQ3.

An interesting question is what the precise role of this author, as a researcher, should be. At one level of ambition, the analysis from the research may reveal a route to improve public policy concerning the English NHS and the adoption of a modified or changed approach to the quasi-market. More realistically the research may solely reveal the boundaries of the author's current understanding of the workings of the English NHS internal market and improve his wider public policy understanding of the existing system and how it performs and is understood. Neither of these two research outcomes, whether personal development or to inform policy, is invalid, and it has been of interest to see, as the research has developed, which of these two outcomes is delivered, or if the outcome becomes more realistically shared somewhere between the two. In addition to this work and his wider roles, the author contributes to the teaching of two master's programmes on health finance policy, and here he has been able to include the discussion around the relevant practitioner-related positions.

The relevance of the research is high. The NHS is undergoing an intense period of change. The need for further improvements in efficiency to deal with: an ageing population; rapid changes to the way NHS could, and should, be delivered; technological improvements that could lead to higher potential costs of treatments; whilst having little opportunity for further increases in funding due largely to the country's overall fiscal position. The central tension in the 2012 Health Act surrounded the role and scope for competition in the NHS. As the then Health Secretary, Lansley (2012: 1) noted:

> In healthcare, the term "competition" is often used pejoratively by vested interests with something to fear from change. But the vast majority of the NHS – including the many world-beating services we have which already compete with other health providers on a global scale – recognise there is nothing to fear from competition.

Figure 3.3 - Research Chronology, the changing English NHS and Changing Research Design

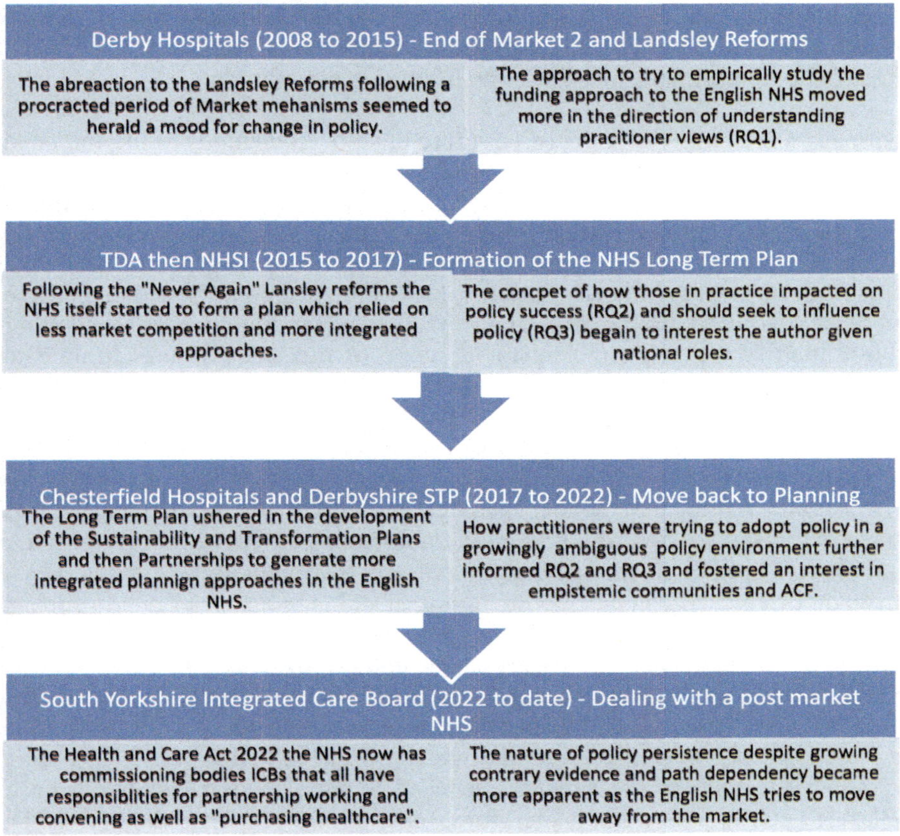

Derby Hospitals (2008 to 2015) - End of Market 2 and Landsley Reforms

The abreaction to the Landsley Reforms following a procracted period of Market mehanisms seemed to herald a mood for change in policy.

The approach to try to empirically study the funding approach to the English NHS moved more in the direction of understanding practitioner views (RQ1).

TDA then NHSI (2015 to 2017) - Formation of the NHS Long Term Plan

Following the "Never Again" Lansley reforms the NHS itself started to form a plan which relied on less market competition and more integrated approaches.

The concpet of how those in practice impacted on policy success (RQ2) and should seek to influence policy (RQ3) begain to interest the author given national roles.

Chesterfield Hospitals and Derbyshire STP (2017 to 2022) - Move back to Planning

The Long Term Plan ushered in the development of the Sustainability and Transformation Plans and then Partnerships to generate more integrated plannign approaches in the English NHS.

How practitioners were trying to adopt policy in a growingly ambiguous policy environment further informed RQ2 and RQ3 and fostered an interest in empistemic communities and ACF.

South Yorkshire Integrated Care Board (2022 to date) - Dealing with a post market NHS

The Health and Care Act 2022 the NHS now has commissioning bodies ICBs that all have responsibilites for partnership working and convening as well as "purchasing healthcare".

The nature of policy persistence despite growing contrary evidence and path dependency became more apparent as the English NHS tries to move away from the market.

The purpose of this research was therefore to evaluate the extent to which the internal market in health has or had a funding environment robust enough to deliver competition, and whether it is deliverable as currently conceived. Also, to see if it has sufficient practitioner support and understanding to achieve this vision associated with this approach. It then sought to develop an approach to understanding how practitioners can appropriately suggest improvements to the existing system.

The research approach adopted sought to steer a course through empirical research and a narrative account of the policy process in health. Bias was to a certain extent inevitable, but was acknowledged and the author reflected on this to ensure that bias was minimised. Although the research aims of the thesis are quite wide, there was a belief that the author will be able to secure quite a high degree of the required engagement from the NHS and stakeholders in order to ensure that the project could access the data and secure participation in the attitudinal research, and then document this to enable the writing of the thesis, and disseminating its findings following completion.

Through the course of the research, there have been changes to the intended methodologies used for the three research aims. As mentioned, when the author was employed in Derby the access to the data associated with the secondary analysis of the publicly available data on hospital performance was not easily accessible to him. Following the author's change of role to go and work at the Trust Development Authority and then NHS Improvement these data became more accessible as did the level of access to senior individuals that the author could attain. Originally, the intended scope of the analysis was limited to hospital provider organisations only. As the data became available for all NHS provider organisations, including mental health and community trusts, this fuller data set was utilised.

The original approach to gaining stakeholder views on the internal market was to use a revised version of a pilot study questionnaire. An opportunity to use and shape a project in which the author was involved via his role with HFMA made it possible to get a much wider range of stakeholder views on the current limitations of the English NHS finance system. This revised approach to the research was therefore co-designed by the author, the data gathered from 203 NHS stakeholders making the findings far more representative than if this element of the research had been undertaken as per the original design. This revised approach was also methodologically preferred based on the growing acknowledgement that the research needed to be more abductive in its approach (Blaikie (2007). The author, therefore, used all the response data from the HFMA/PwC report, and its surveys; trying to better identify the qualitative motivations of senior staff, and giving a much broader body of evidence, than if this research had been solely performed quantitively, by the author alone.

The final selection of the stakeholder group to discuss the findings of the research, became self-selecting, via the author's participation in the HFMAs Policy and Research Committee. The author considered it sensible to use a specialist forum to which he had access to discuss the research as the proposed stakeholder group. This made the research ethics easier, as all the participants were willing to participate in the required discussion as part of their role on the Committee. This Committee itself has a good spread of participants, from Scotland, Wales and Northern Ireland and each element of the English system (Department of Health, NHSE, NHSI). The Committee is specifically composed to have this representative spread of stakeholders, between providers of different types (community services, acute and mental health), commissioners, and participation beyond the English NHS to the wider UK. A lone academic or practitioner-researcher mobilising this sort of stakeholder group to discuss and influence the research and discuss findings would find it exceptionally hard to construct a group which balanced different perspectives on the UK NHS. Using the group which has a stated aim of influencing policy also assists greatly with the action research aims.

Although there are doubtless limitations of this approach to the study contained within this thesis, as with all social science, surrounding the difficulties of identifying cause and effect and the right approach to research design, the author has been very fortunate in being able to exploit his insider position. The "role-based emergent opportunism" approach has:

1. enabled access to a broader set of data than was originally intended for the first research objective.

2. enabled the generation of a much wider set of stakeholder view data than was originally intended, via shaping the work of a national report on NHS finance, in which the author has been involved. This changed approach meets the original research objectives, but has a wider reach and has engaged with 203 NHS finance stakeholders seeking their more authentic views on the internal market.

3. delivered a ready-made representative stakeholder group to discuss the findings of the first two areas of research to meet the third research aim, with all participants volunteering for further discussions on the project, if and as required.

3.9 Health Policy and Key Analytical Themes within the Study

The following is an attempt to try and orientate the reader to the various health policy and key analytical themes contained within the thesis and where they are explored within this document. The matrix in Table 3.3 notes seven key themes of the research and was derived by mapping the overall content of the thesis into key conceptual strands. The table notes eight different main analytical key themes with the research including:

1. Social and Cultural Reproduction and "Worldview" – which notes the nature of knowledge in this area of research and points towards its relatively subjective nature.

2. New Public Management – which is asserted as the academic foundation of the internal market policy.

3. Health Public Policy and Politics – which addresses the inter-dependency between political ideas and public policy to support those ideas.

4. Policy Implementation – which explores the concepts around policy implementation and top-down versus bottom-up views of policy determination and adoption.

5. Narrative Accounts of Health Policy – which note the more subjective and narrative accounts in the exploration and determination of health policy.

6. Nature of Healthcare System Value – which describes the aims of healthcare systems.

7. Abductive and Action Research – which gives an approach to try and form conclusions from subjective knowledge and opinion and then change policy and approach as a result.

8. Insider and Practitioner Knowledge in NHS Finance – note the role of practitioner research and explains where this can be used to best effect.

Table 3.3 - Matrix of Health Policy and Resource Key Analytical Themes

Theories/ Literature Sources	Health and analytical key themes	Topic Impact on thesis	Professional insights and reflection	Place in thesis	Outcomes in research and learning
Cresswell (2009) Bruyn (1963)	***Social and cultural reproduction and Worldview***	Explores practitioner standpoint as a key part of research process to develop alternatives.	Acknowledges fully the subjectivity of concepts such as the NHS internal market. Shapes the need for abductive research and the need to try and influence views.	3.2/3.3/3.4 5.3/5.4 8.1	Notes and reflects on objective versus subjective views of reality and questions standing of attitudinal and action research.
Hayek (1944) Niskanen (1971) Tullock (2000)	***New Public Management***	Tries to examine public policy from a political New Right perspective, that originated criticisms of state provision.	Traces the political and public policy rationale for the approach to experimenting with an internal market in health.	2.3 8.1	Seeks to understand original underpinning of quasi market policy to better understand academic and policy perspective which may have generated "Working for Patients" (1989).
Klein (2013) Bagot (2007) Paton C. (2016)	***Health Public Policy and Politics***	Gives different accounts of the interplay between politics and policy which provides understanding of contextual factors	Developed thinking around the interconnectedness between politics, policy and then the approach to changing or amending existing funding mechanisms or structures.	2.1/2.2/2.3/2.5 4.1 5.3	Contextualises the author's practitioner perspective on the nature of the policy environment and its political antecedent, building, and giving permission for the thesis' own narrative account.
Wildavsky (1992) Lipsky (2010)	***Policy Implementation***	Notes different views of the way in which policy is determined and adopted.	Gave clarity to the approach associated with the role of practitioners in the development of policy and different perspectives on policy implementation	3.2 5.1	Examines approach to policy implementation, which is then specifically explored, and findings made, in the action research phase.

Table 3.3 - Continued

Theories/ Literature Sources	Health and analytical key themes	Topic Impact on thesis	Professional insights and reflection	Place in thesis	Outcomes in research and learning
Tuohy (1999) Marmor (2007)	*Narrative Accounts of Health Policy*	Gives a subject area specific set of accounts of the way in which health policy has been described then practice set up and ultimately adopted.	Assimilation of different perspectives on health and events with the formation of NHS and current approach to policy and structures	2.1/2.2/2.3 2.4/2.7 5.1 8.1	Validated the approach to the author's own narrative account and enabled an approach to examining the findings of the HFMA/PWC report. Validated approach to bolder and broader conclusions.
Mintzberg (2017) Gray (2017) Fox (2018)	*Nature of Healthcare System Value*	How do we define and understand value in healthcare systems and the NHS	To what extent do we have agreement and clarity on the way in which we should measure and assess high value health services.	1.2 2.4 2.6	Gave the author additional insight into the extent to which a market could deliver these policy goals
Blaikie (2007) Hart and Bond (1995)	*Abductive and Action Research*	Abductive design for qualitive views AR questionnaire, Power and Influence, Force Field Analysis	Clearly described the need to emphasise the subjective knowledge of practitioners and the need for the research to try and address and be a catalyst for change	3.1/3.4 5.2 6.2	Gave a framework for the approach and the findings from both the attitudinal and action research, noting dissent but need for change.
Drake and Heath (2011) Wilkinson (2000)	*Insider and Practitioner Knowledge in NHS Finance*	Practitioner Narrative Accounts, Regression Analysis of Provider Performance	Costing and Pricing in the NHS Provider and Commissioner Financial Management Trust, STP and NHS Financial Structures	2.5 3.1 4.2/4.3/4.5 7.2/7.3.	Enabled and gave permission for the equal standing of practitioner views, through the research design and the conclusions and recommendations.

CHAPTER 4

FINDINGS - DO FINANCE PRACTITIONERS BELIEVE NHS FUNDING COULD RUN A MARKET?

This chapter looks at how healthcare provider organisations are funded: looking at the pre-pandemic financial performance of English NHS Providers and the overall English NHS. It seeks to answer the question as to whether the funding mechanisms could ever have been sufficient to deliver an internal market, in the opinion of the practitioners, in the field, who implement and observe the policy. It uses regression analysis performed by the author and tests the findings from that analysis in the Policy and Research Committee of the HFMA. It uses the HFMA Policy and Research Committee as a sample of practitioners, to see if they believe that the way in which the NHS is funded could run a market.

If the internal market were to work, it would need an adequate payment system to organisations. This payment system needs to be able to deliver the appropriate exit to the NHS provider market, of an individual inefficient provider (or some inefficient services within providers). However, due to the inability of individual providers to deliver the required healthcare within the overall pricing system, delivered through the NHS tariff for services, there were several organisational deficits in the system in 2016/17 (and mechanisms to fund them) than a market could or would allow. 2016/17 can be seen as a typical pre-pandemic year with an NHS provider deficit position, balanced by other parts of the DHSC in surplus, which is described further in this chapter.

As described in Section 3.8, this chapter uses quantitative regression analysis to identify the correlations between good and bad financial performance in English NHS provider organisations, and a series of selected independent variables. The independent variable was selected by the author and then their selection checked with the HFMA Policy and Research Committee. It was based on available secondary data, (which the author had insider access to in the correct form to more easily enable the collation and the analysis). The results of the analysis were then discussed with the HFMA Policy and Research Committee. This data, which was made available to the author by the Directors of Finance of NHSE and NHSI. The author had to manipulate and analyse this data in Excel and then discuss this analysis with the HFMA Policy and Research Committee to form a conclusion on the first research question.

4.1 The Nature of English NHS Healthcare Organisation Funding

As earlier noted, the thesis has descoped the question of whether there is sufficient funding going into the overall English NHS system. The pre-pandemic financial position of the NHS is worthy of note as the starting point of this chapter, though. The DoH in England had a budget and spent £115.6 bn in 2016/17. This section next draws heavily on a National Audit Office (2018) report on NHS finances.

The pre-pandemic NHS provider position was in significant underlying financial deficit. There would be very many providers now who should have been subject to "exit" and the failure regime, based on their financial performance. The reported deficit in 2016/17, following the receipt of a relatively new element of funding, the Sustainability and Transformation funding (STF), was a deficit of £791m. However, if the STF is removed, then the overall deficit position for the whole NHS provider sector was £2.7bn in the 2016/17 financial year. This was the last set of fully audited accounts data that was available at the time of undertaking this element of the research.

> Key Facts Associated with Current NHS Provider Performance
>
> £791m – the combined deficit of NHS trusts and NHS foundation trust in 2016/17
> £1.8bn - sustainability and transformation funding for trusts in 2016/17
> £2.7bn - extra revenue funding given to trusts as interest-bearing loans in 2016/17 (NAO (2018); 3).

It is evident from these figures, that the financial position of the overall provider sector is in a somewhat difficult position. There were insufficient resources in aggregate flowing to the providers of NHS treatment and care to deliver the care being provided by them. At this point, it is important to pose the question – "Why was the NHS not overspent overall and breaking the Parliamentary vote associated with the cash limit, given to it by the Treasury and Parliament?". The NAO described this via other elements of the overall Department of Health budgets.

> Key Findings Associated with Overall NHS financial performance
>
> 1. In 2016/17, NHS commissioners and trusts reported a combined surplus of £111 million, not including adjustments needed to report against departments' budget for day-to-day resources and Administration costs.

2. The NHS achieved its overall surplus in 2016/17 by planning a series of measures to rebalance its finances, some of which have restricted the money available for longer-term transformation.

3. In 2016/17, the national bodies gave £4.1 billion in financial support to trusts outside of service contracts with commissioners which does not support effective planning.

4. The financial deficit position of the trust sector significantly reduced in 2016/17, but failure to achieve its target position has limited the resources available to transform services and built financial pressure for future years.

5. Clinical Commissioning Groups and trusts are significantly reliant on one-off measures to deliver savings, posing significant risks to financial sustainability in the future. (NAO, 2018: 5)

Essentially, the provider deficits were offset by commissioning underspends, taking the money earmarked for a redesign in the NHS's Sustainability and Transformation Plan funding, and the revenue deficit was addressed via reduced capital spending. As a direct consequence of the funding regime, the NAO made a series of recommendations to address the immediate issues of the NHS finance regime which continued into 2017/18 and 2018/19.

NAO Recommendations on Value for Money in the English NHS System

a) The Department, NHS England and NHS Improvement should, within the confines of current legislation, move further and faster towards system-wide incentives and regulation.

b) The Department, NHS England and NHS Improvement should assess how funding currently available from the sustainability and transformation fund can best support trusts beyond 2018/19.

c) The Department, NHS England and NHS Improvement should assess whether the various financial flows and management approaches they use are working as intended and take remedial action if necessary.

d) The Department and NHS England need to gain greater clarity over the fundamental financial pressures in the trust sector when allocating funding to clinical commissioning groups and directly to Trusts.

e) NHS England and NHS Improvement should continue to align their resources and regulatory functions to better support local partnerships.

f) The Department, working with NHS England and NHS Improvement, should set out when the committed capital investment for transformation and backlogs of the central maintenance will be made available.

g) NHS England and NHS Improvement should give those local partnerships making the slowest progress sufficient financial support and opportunities to transform services. (NAO (2018); 6).

These recommendations are broadly congruent with the recommendations made in earlier sources, namely more integrated oversight and management for the whole system, along with more specific financial recommendations, related to (i) the overall financial system in the English NHS, (ii) the use of the Sustainability and Transformation Fund (which had become used, since its inception in 2015/16, as a 'bail-out fund' for the deficit in the provider organisations), and (iii) a more appropriate approach to access required capital funding.

The nature of healthcare delivery is exceptionally complex, and the dissent on the appropriateness and/or adequacy of an internal market is at issue. Either the purchaser/provider split can be made to work with the correct amount of skill and/or will, or it cannot. Porter and Tiesberg's (2006) view is that the inherent bureaucracy of the English NHS was never skilled enough or had the will to deliver the benefits that competition could offer. There may also be the claim that politicians and policymakers did not have the necessary fortitude that would enable the market and competition to flourish (i.e., forcing an individual hospital or health care organisation or services to close).

Alternatively, it could be that the market mechanism required to enable a fully functional market, categorised by exit, at the point of failure, was never the intention or within the scope of policy design. Market failure has perhaps never been an overt policy objective of each accretive piece of internal market policy and legislation. Perhaps, without this being overt in the design and policy intent, the actors or street-level bureaucrats in the NHS system have never taken the policy seriously enough to enact the legislation to get to the logical consequence of the internal market.

The author's position on this, however, is that an internal market in the English NHS never had, and never could have, a pricing and reimbursement mechanism which could incentivise the right behaviour, even if the policy aims had been desirable. The integrated nature of healthcare meant that the purchaser/provider split, as conceived of in the English system, was never adequate to deliver allocative efficiency, unit cost efficiency or market-based 'X-efficiency' (Leibenstein, 1966) which is considered by economists as the efficiency which is derived from the competition in a market. The author's position on this issue is compared with other practitioners' views in Chapter 5.

4.2 The Costing and Pricing of NHS Treatment and Care in England

Of particular interest is the extent to which the specified services, which are costed and priced in the English NHS system to deliver the internal market system, are adequate to either differentiate between, (a) good and bad provider organisation financial performance, or (b) get as far as being able to give good price signals to deliver improvements in care by certain providers entering or exiting elements of service, or (c) ultimately leading to the failure of poor performing services or organisations. The commodifying and calculating myth (#5), as described by Mintzberg (2017), is highly prevalent in the English NHS system in the opinion of the author. National prices are set through the annual process called Reference Costs. All providers in the system take their overall costs of provision and each year, they divide those total costs into a series of nationally determined and specified activity measures. In hospitals, these activity measures include:

i. Emergency department attendances (grouped by what sorts of investigations they had whilst in the emergency department)

ii. Outpatient attendance both new and follow-up/review, tends to be costed at the specialty level, e.g., dermatology or gastroenterology. There is also a subcategory of outpatient procedures, where sub-day or day case type work may occur in an outpatient context.

iii. Day case attendances (which tend to be for minor surgical procedures, clinical investigation or other procedures) are then grouped based on the clinical coding of the diagnosis of the patients and the procedure(s) which are undertaken on them.

iv. Planned/elective inpatient treatments, where patients stay in the hospital overnight; for planned procedures, following a clinical review, usually requiring surgery. These activities are then also grouped based on their clinical coding of the diagnosis of the patients and the procedure(s) which are undertaken on them.

v. Non-Elective or Emergency inpatient treatments are then grouped in the same way that day cases and planned inpatients are.

Within the admitted patient care types, (iv. and v., above), the grouping that delivers the activity type, based on the diagnostic and procedure codes, given to the hospital episodes results in a grouping to a Healthcare Resource Group (HRG) that is individually costed. All these HRGs based on their diagnostic coding will have categories with or without complications. The "with complications" HRGs tend to have higher costs and consequently higher prices.

vi. Also, within the HRGs for inpatients, there is an additional payment that may be due, due to excess bed days, beyond a nationally determined number of days of stay, in the hospital, which attracts a cost and therefore prices per day.

vii. There are also several further activity currencies nationally determined such as haemo-dialysis sessions or patients on other forms of renal replacement therapy, for example, which are nationally costed and priced.

viii. Finally, there are categories of treatment where there are no nationally set currencies and therefore prices which are subject to local specification and the pricing within each organisation and system.

Latterly the costing and pricing model has been used by the HRG system/approach to determine which of the areas of clinical work, particularly for hospitals, is being commissioned by the CCGs or specialist commissioning, via NHSE. Relatively common clinical work is commissioned by the CCGs, and unusual or more specialist nature work is commissioned nationally, via NHS England.

The services and costs which fall out of the treatment and care definitions in the Reference Cost submission (viii) are then commissioned by either the CCGs or NHSE using local prices (different for each Trust). Intensive care medicine and stays in intensive care units have local prices charged to both the CCGs and NHSE depending on the nature of the patient stays.

There are then some services and costs in providers that are not borne by either NHS commissioner, such as private patient work, work funded charitably, or education and training costs, that fall outside Reference Cost activity and cost definitions, completely. Within the funding model of the English NHS there is therefore a hugely complex series of products and prices, which are either set nationally or locally.

The core funding for each NHS provider organisation was, up to the pandemic, therefore determined via an annual national process of Reference Costs, where each provider submits its overall cost data to NHS Improvement. These cost data were then used to determine the national prices, which were contractually bound between commissioners and providers in the national pricing system, which determined the average prices for each of the listed activities above to determine the national prices. Other services had locally determined activities and prices.

An entire thesis could be written on the national costing and pricing system. The author used to chair the HFMA subcommittee on the National Payment System, which provided a reference group of practitioners, to try and advise, at the time, NHSE (responsible for the currency definitions), NHSI (responsible for the pricing methodology) and NHS Digital (responsible for the HRG grouping methodology), on how to improve the system. All these functions are now performed by NHSE, following the 2022 merger of NHS Digital and NHS Improvement with it. The National Payment System or Payments by Results system, is shown in Figure 4.1 and is defined as:

> Payment by Results (PbR) is the tariff-based payment system that has transformed the way funding flows around the NHS in England... PbR began in a limited way, with national tariffs for 15 HRGs in 2003-04 and 48 HRGs in 2004-05. The first NHS foundation trust (FT) applicants moved to the full PbR system in 2005-06 and other NHS trusts in 2006-07. PbR now represents over 60% of acute hospital income and about one-third of primary care trust (PCT) budgets. (DoH, 2012: 4)

Figure 4.1 - Department of Health (2007) Schematic - Introduction of Payments by Results

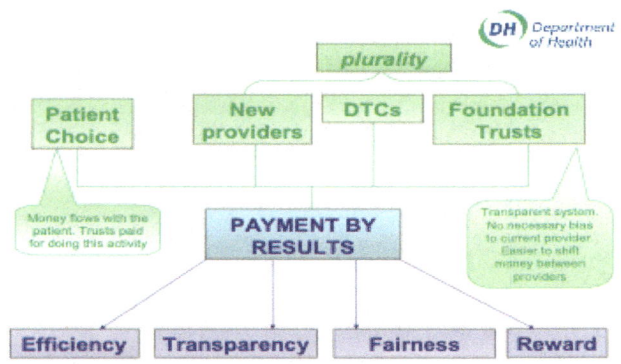

Some immediate observations, by the author, on the Payments by Results policy include:

- Payments by Results actively incentivised clinical work to be undertaken, particularly in an acute context. Hospital income is generated by the volume of clinical activity completed.
- The definitions of the clinical work undertaken are not frequently refreshed and do not quickly allow for innovation away from the historically used definitions.
- Particularly, for example, if a care provider is good at stepping down non-elective care from inpatient to day-case to outreach care, resulting in a costlier and sicker cohort of patients being admitted to the hospital as inpatients, it is unclear if the HRG grouping system and average cost pricing would satisfactorily reimburse for this.
- The same argument as that made immediately above could also be made associated with the elective pathway and organisations that step down care from inpatient to day-case to outpatient procedure, resulting in the residual work at inpatient and day-case levels being more complex than the average.
- The extent to which the definition of the clinical work described in the Payment by Results system truly describes hospital activity that is both iso-resource (should cost the same) and clinically meaningful (a claim made by the system) is contested by practitioners.
- A further unintended consequence of the PbR system could also be seen to be the fact that acute hospital NHS services and definitions tended to be covered by this approach and services in other parts of the system are not. GP services, community services, social care, services and mental health services are not covered by the fee-for-service model. Funding may therefore have been screwed towards the hospital sector via this approach.

Figure 4.2 – Author's Own Diagram - Approach to Improvement within the Hospital Setting

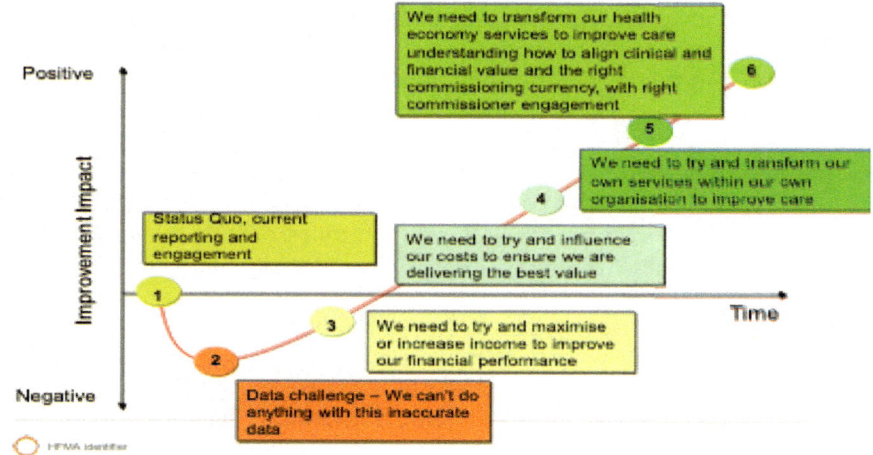

The author has used Figure 4.2 on the Payment by Results system when teaching NHS finance in hospitals and wider settings. The j-curve, which is illustrative, notes that the initial response to the Payment by Results construct, once it is understood, gives rise to the need to manage provider finances in a particular way. The model for payment requires understanding and data (at point 2) noting the complexity of the reimbursement mechanism described above, followed by the understanding of the fact that the more clinical work under-taken the more the hospital will get paid (at point 3), before focusing on the actual costs of delivery and improving them where possible (at point 4). Beyond these initial stages, we then get further into more complex discussions around financial management and service delivery, such as: how we change the way we deliver services which may negatively impact hospital income (at point 5); before we may then move on to discuss whole system financial improvement, (at point 6); which should be the overall aim of NHS financial management to deliver a high value health and social care service.

4.3 Practitioner Views on English NHS Provider Financial Performance

The available academic literature on the overall approach to funding the English NHS system is somewhat sparse, in terms of how it is administered and the views within the system. The author, as part of his role as an HFMA trustee, is exceptionally keen on practitioner research on health policy and finance. As well as working on this doctorate, the author has also supported work which has developed the current HFMA qualifications to the master's level. As part of this work, there is now more practitioner research on health finance, and a research project is a key component of the master's level qualification. The author is hoping that the HFMA qualification will enable a far broader strand of practitioner research in health finance. Currently, there is little specific academic literature on healthcare finance. The access which the author's role has given him is considerable and points to a tension between the information needed to research health finance and the difficulty of individual researchers to access it. Also, a detailed knowledge of the concepts involved, coupled with a public sector-chartered accountancy qualification, makes the analysis here an insider's view of the overall funding system in health. These factors pose several challenges for the researcher-practitioner, namely, how to evidence the importance and the adequacy of the work undertaken and how to explain it.

Earlier in the chapter, using the NAO work, the overall financial performance of the English NHS was described. This section of the research looks at the financial performance of individual providers within the NHS provider sector, to try and establish if there is a correlation between financial performance and independent variables, that might be causing financial performance. It uses bi-variate regression analysis performed, using Microsoft Excel, which was used given the availability of, and familiarity with, this application to the author. Excel has a graphing function which can also perform r^2 analysis, generating lines of best fit the correlation co-efficients reported here.

In statistics, linear regression is an approach to modelling the relationship between a dependent variable y and an explanatory variable denoted x. The case of examining one explanatory variable is called bivariate regression. Bivariate regression analysis can therefore help with identifying the relationships between two variables. In an experiment where the dependent variable has a perfect linear relationship with the explanatory variable the coefficient of determination, (r^2), or "goodness of fit", would be 1.00 or 100%. This is described by Gujarati (1988: 68) as 'the regression context, r^2 ...provides an overall measure of the extent to which the variation in one variable determines the variation in the other'. In social science, where there are lots of variables in complex systems, there are very few experiments, correlations or causal relationships which result in such a perfect linear relationship being established.

The data used for this analysis were collated from sources from DHSC, and specifically by the Directors of Finance of NHSE and NHSI, by the author. Data for each of the 238 NHS provider organisations and each of their variables used for the bivariate and then multivariate regression analysis. Some of the data mapping to each of the providers was more complex than others, such as the CCG mapping to each provider, but this was performed using the author's knowledge of the NHS and the NHS finance regime. The data is summarised in Table 4.1, which shows the minimum, maximum, mean and standard deviation of each of the variables. The table also shows a short summary of the potential correlation hypothesis, in the view of the author, that was then shared and tested with the HFMA Policy and Research Committee. In the stakeholder/ focus group/action research stage of the project, described in Chapter 6, the analysis was described using Figure 4.1 as a starting point to elicit reflections on the current English NHS finding approach. Figure 4.1 shows the dependent variables used in the regression against provider organisation surplus/deficit as a proportion of turnover (Y) versus the independent variables, listed below, (X1 to X12.)

Table 4.1 - Regression Analysis Variables on Healthcare Organisation Financial Performance:

Variable	Min	Max	Mean	SD	Hypothesis
Deficit £m pre STF	21.4	-115.3	-11.4	18.4	{NB £21.4 is a surplus!}
Deficit % (y)	5.32	-23.4	-3.23	4.95	{NB 5.32% is a surplus!}
Turnover £M (x1)	22.4	1,302	268	191	Larger more resilience
RCI (x2)	77.9	153	100	10.4	"Efficient" more surplus
RC as % Turnover (x3)	37.5	99.9	78.9	10.5	Diversification helps
%£ from 1° CCG (x4)	0.02	97.1	41.3	36.5	Interdependency +ve/-ve?
CCG Deficit £m (x5)	32	-120	0	21	Win/Lose – CGG fine, Trust not
CCG DfT % (x6)	-5	30	0	4.4	Less funding a problem
MFF (x7)	0.93	1.20	1.00	0.06	Higher MFF, surplus easier
NHSE % (x8)	0	73.7	14.5	14.3	Specialist "easier"
PFI Cap/Turnover % (x9)	0	114.1	9.2	20	PFI a problem
Ed/Research % (x10)	0	65.3	4.4	5.6	Better to have more
CQC Rating (x11)	1	4	2.53	0.7	Quality costs
ED Performance (x12)	72.37	100	88.9	6.2	Performance Costs

Within the overall deficit position of the English NHS Providers described by the NAO, the maximum surplus made by one organisation, the pre-Sustainability and Transformation Fund, was £21.4m. The worst deficit within an individual NHS organisation was £115.3m. The average deficit for all providers, including those in surplus, was £11.4m. The turnovers of NHS Provider organisations ranged from the smallest Trust having a turnover of £22.4m, to the largest having a turnover of £1.3bn. The average turnover for an NHS provider organisation was £268m. When expressed as a proportion of turnover, the largest surplus was 5.32%, the biggest deficit was 23.4%, and the average deficit (including surpluses) expressed as a percentage of overall NHS provider turnover was 3.23%. The deficit as a proportion of turnover was used as the dependent variable (Y) as the absolute size of surplus/deficit is correlated to the size of the NHS provider organisation. Each of the hypotheses between the variables is explained further in Section 4.4.

Before dealing with the regression analysis and looking at patterns of what may or may not be correlated to deficits, it is perhaps worth pausing and considering a couple of methodological points. First, what is or is not included in these reported surplus/deficit numbers; and the second was 16/17 a typical financially performing year for the NHS provider sector, prior to the pandemic, and how constant is the distribution of those surpluses and deficits year on year (i.e. do they vary widely across providers each year or do they remain relatively constant across the provider base).

The statutorily reported financial position for the annual accounts for NHS providers in 2016/17 probably understates the overall underlying deficit position of the provider sector. It is however difficult to pick out individual transactions which are buoying up individual providers and the sector's overall financial performance, which are one-off. So, for example, individual asset sales which generate a profit on disposal will be included in the numbers. Also, technical items which see the revaluation of the asset values of the Trusts, reducing the Trust's Public Dividend Capital costs (the circular flow of funds charged to the Department of Health for Trusts holding assets), which was a system which started back in 1991, when the idea of self-governing hospitals first required them to have a balance sheet, will be included in the reported surplus/deficit numbers. There may be other one-off benefits included in the reported numbers. Therefore, although the overall reported position is an overall sector deficit for providers of £2.7bn, the author is aware that national NHSI estimates of the recurrent deficit for the sector, without these one-off impacts were estimated at around £4.0bn.

The changing deficit position for the provider sector is well documented in the NAO report. The overall net provider position in the English NHS reported surpluses of £513m, £483m, and £592m in 2010/11, 2011/12 and 2012/13, respectively. 2013/14 saw a move to a small net deficit position of £91m, with a move to a more significant deficit position in 2014/15 of £859m. Since then, the provider deficit has bottomed out at a relatively constant (if slightly deteriorating) set of values of £2,447m in 2015/16, followed by a deficit before the provider sector receipt of the Sustainability and Transformation Fund of £2,587m in 2016/17. The actual reported position for the provider sector in 2017/18 was a £2,869m deficit (a post-STF position of £1,086m, with £1,783m

STF applied). Therefore, there has been a change in the overall reported position of the provider sector in the period 2015/16 to 2017/18, as shown in Figure 4.3, adopting 2016/17 as the base year for the regression analysis work should be representative of the pre-pandemic funding approach.

Figure 4.3 – NAO (2018) Surplus/Deficits of Trusts 2010/11 to 2017/18

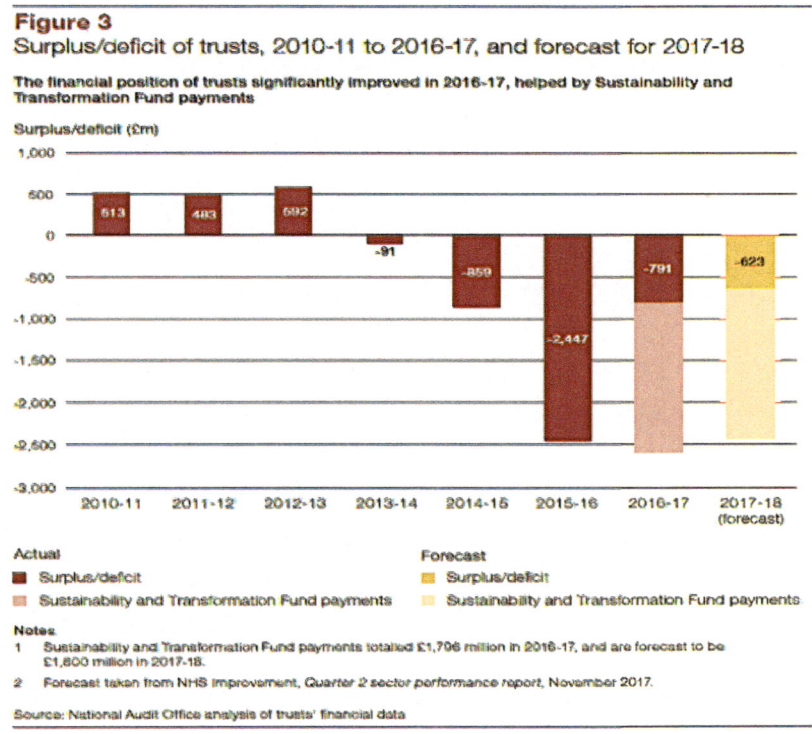

Also, it is worth checking whether the overall deficit position is constant across NHS provider organisations or whether it moves around within them. To evidence the relative constancy across providers, analysis has been performed comparing the 2017/18 surplus deficit outturn data with the same data for 2016/17. It shows a correlation of financial performance of r-squared 58%, as shown in Figure 4.4. Therefore, although there is some degree of financial volatility within the overall provider financial performance, the analysis of the 232 providers, (which had common organisational forms in 16/17 and 17/18 – there tend to be some mergers and changes each year) shows a reasonable correlation of financial performance year on year.

It is also worth noting at this point that the deficit position across the NHS is not evenly split either by type of Trust (acute, ambulance, community, mental health or specialist) or regionally (there were four reporting regions with NHSE/NHSI regional offices (London, Midlands and East, North and South). Broadly defined, the financial challenge from a deficit perspective was an acute (i.e., hospital) sector problem and there was a greater financial problem in the Midlands and East when compared with the then three other NHS regions. There are now seven regions that oversee the work of the ICBs.

Figure 4.4 - Deficit position of Trusts 2016/17 compared to 2017/18

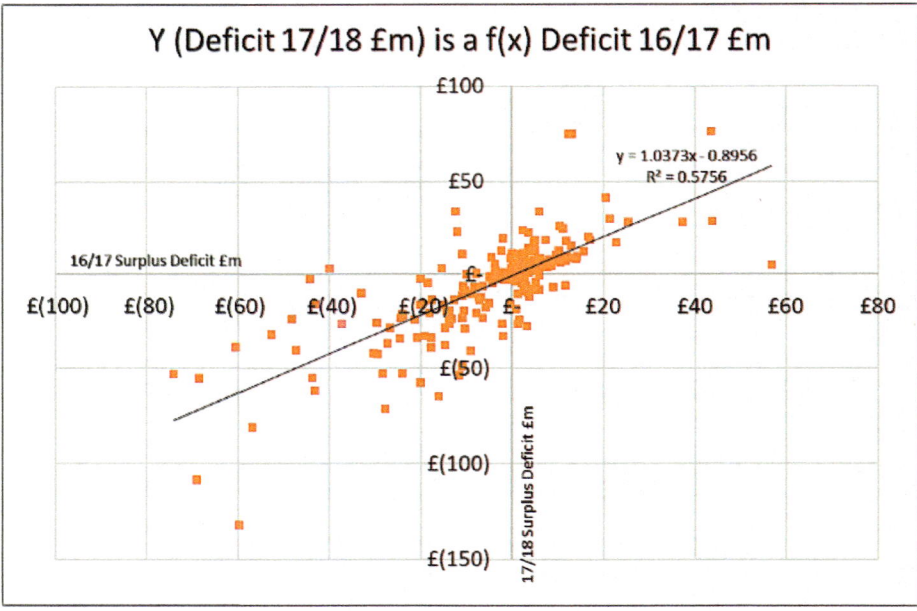

4.4 Bivariate Regression Analysis into causal factors for health provider financial performance 2016/17

4.4.1 Financial Performance versus Turnover

The first variable analysed looked to find a correlation between surplus deficit/and the sizes of the NHS organisations themselves. When expressed as a proportion of turnover, the largest surplus was 5.32% (Clatterbridge a specialist cancer centre); the biggest deficit was 23.4% (North Cumbria Trust). The pre-regression expectation from this analysis was that there may have been a negative correlation between deficits and size, with larger trusts able to cope with the nature of the payment system and other financial issues and having the ability to share their Trust overheads across a wider cost base. This does not seem to be the case, however, as the correlation between size and deficit is negative; and the r2 associated with the correlation is a statistically insignificant 0.18%. Visually, it is not possible to see a pattern in the distribution of the data.

Figure 4.5 - Regression 1 - Deficit percentage of Trusts 2016/17 compared to Trust turnover.

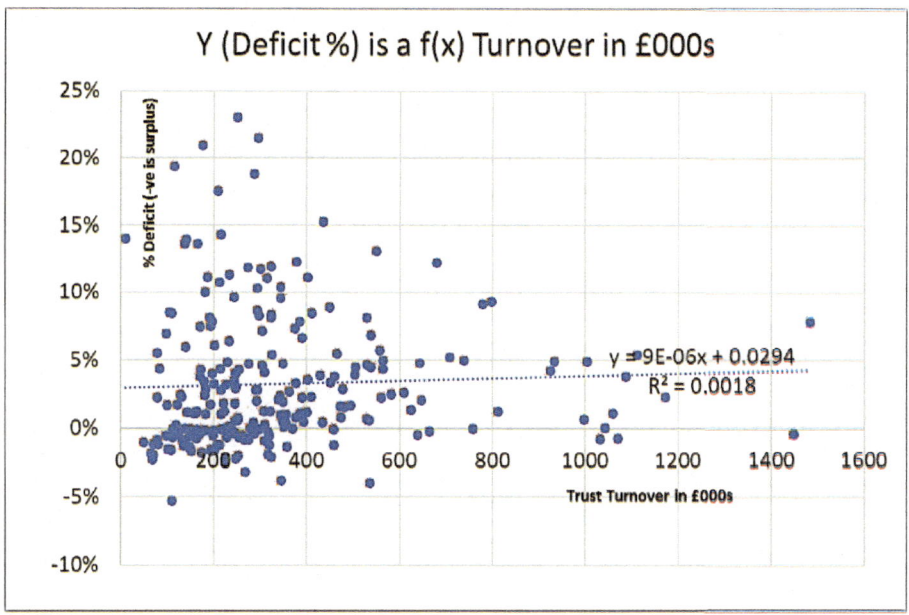

4.4.2 Financial Performance versus Reference Cost Index

The second variable analysed looked at the correlation between surplus/deficit and reference cost index of each individual trust. As part of the reference cost process, each year, each Trust has a reference cost index calculated for it, associated with the overall unit cost efficiency. All the activities included in the Reference Cost submission are given a resource weighting to generate a Trust-wide volume of output. This is then divided into the overall costs of the Trust to give a relative resource measure of unit cost efficiency. If a Trust has an average cost for its outputs it has a Reference Cost Index (RCI) of 100. If unit costs are ten per cent over average, it will have an RCI of 110. If their unit costs are 10% below average an RCI of 90.

The minimum reference cost index in the English NHS organisations is 77.90 (Pennine Care, a non-acute provider), and the highest reference cost is 153.09 (Camden and Islington Trust, another non-acute provider). As already noted, however, community trusts tended to use local prices, so those two Trusts may not to see a surplus/deficit in the anticipated way. Everything else being equal, one would expect to see a correlation between those with a low RCI, and those in surplus. This assumes that the prices are appropriate and the wider determinants of financial health for NHS provider organisations do not have an undue impact on financial performance. The national tariff pricing system sets the prices based on the average reference costs of providers. The RCI is a measure of that very efficiency.

Figure 4.6 – Regression 2 – Deficit percentage of Trusts compared to Reference Cost Index

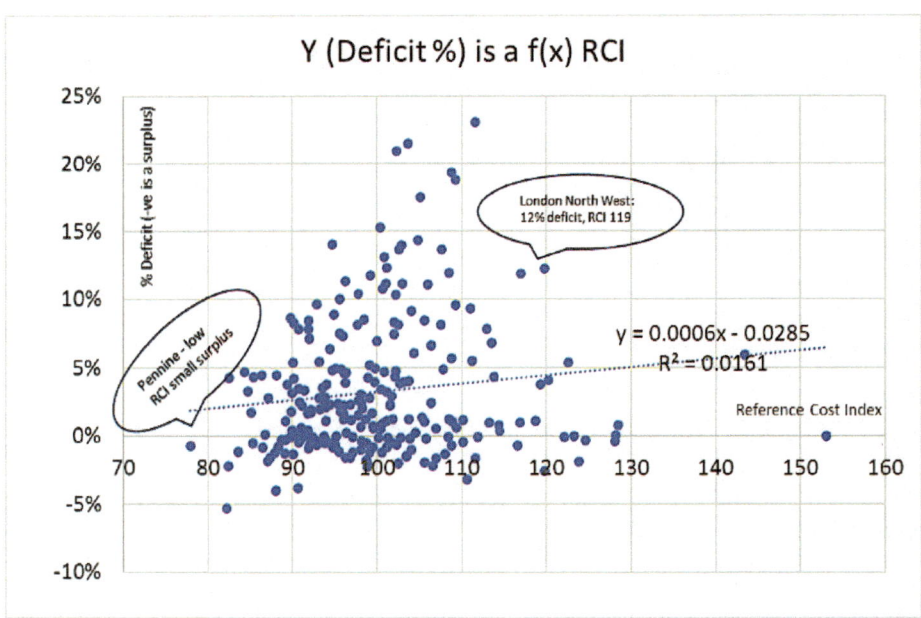

The results of this analysis were particularly perplexing. London North West Trust with an RCI of 119 was delivering a 12% deficit, and Clatterbridge with an RCI of 82.2 was delivering a healthy surplus. These two results adhere to the proposed hypothesis, elsewhere there was wide variation between the relationship of surplus or deficit and the Reference Cost Index. There was an expected positive correlation between deficit and higher RCI, but there was a relatively low r2 of 1.61%. So perplexing was this result that the analysis was re-performed on the acute Trusts only, where there is perhaps slightly less contention and variation on the activity definitions, but even after only using these 137 acute Trusts a positive correlation was found and a higher but still relatively low r2 of 8.49%.

4.4.3 Financial Performance versus Reference Cost/Turnover

The third variable analysed was Reference Costs as a proportion of overall turnover. This is, in essence, a measure of how diversified away from standard treatment and care various healthcare organisations are. The average proportion of turnover within reference costs was 78.90%. The minimum 37.54% was Cornwall Partnership Trust which does much of its work for local government, the highest was 99.87% North Essex Partnership FT. Here there was a more significant positive correlation, with an r2 of 34.5%. A conclusion that can sensibly be drawn from this data is that the more diversified a Trust was the less funding it needed from the core NHS service funding, and the more correlated that is with surpluses.

Figure 4.7 – Regression 3 – Deficit percentage compared to Reference Cost Submission Total

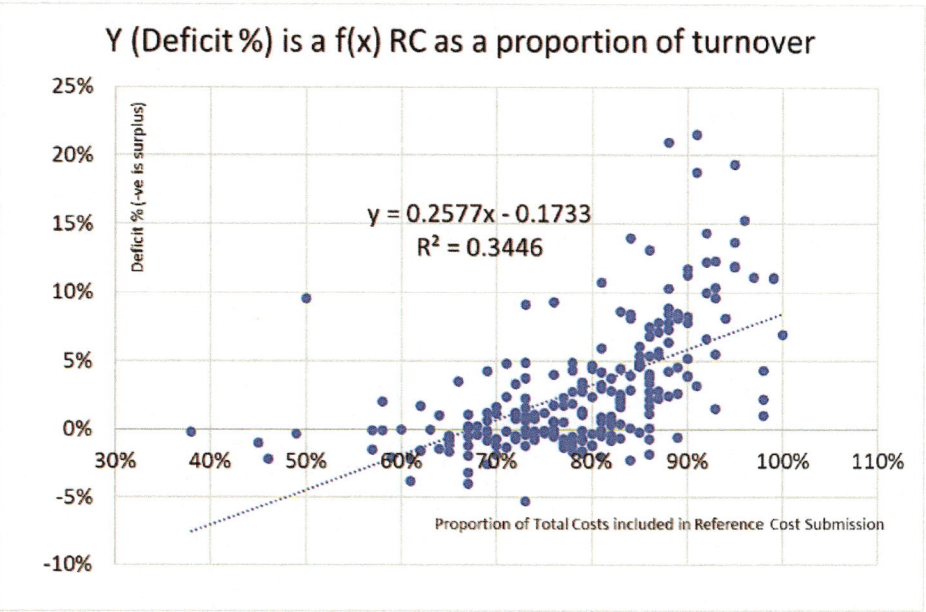

4.4.4 Financial Performance versus Income from main CCG

The next variable used is related to the proportion of the provider's income that previously came from its main CCG. The relationships between provider organisations and their commissioners were many and varied. Some providers had a close one-to-one relationship, with most/all income coming from one commissioner. Some tertiary referral centres had many commissioner relationships and treated patients from a much broader catchment area. Tertiary work is commissioned by NHS England, for work that was defined as specialist commissioning. It was unclear prior to this analysis whether a higher degree of interdependency between commissioners and providers would give rise to an enhanced surplus or deficit position. At one level a cosier monopoly/ monopsony relationship may have given rise to less commissioning challenge, or more mature relationships, so may be positive. Or, this could be negative, if the CCG was under financial distress itself, or its allocation had a high negative Distance from Target. At another level, a low relationship may have given rise to easier commissioning relationships for providers on issues such as non-tariff pricing or other matters, as the provider may have been able to exploit a more monopolistic position for certain services.

Figure 4.8 – Regression 4 – Deficit percentage compared to proportion of income from main CCG.

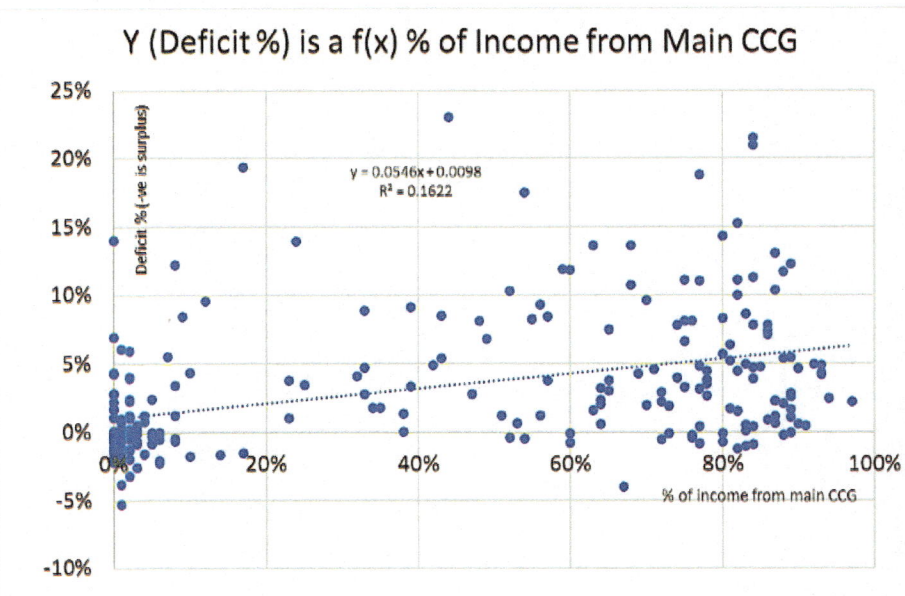

The results of this analysis were of interest. The mean level of income from host CCG for all Trusts was 41.28%. There was a cluster of Trusts, predominantly specialist and tertiary centres which had a percentage of Trust income from the main commissioner as low as 0.02%. The highest income to a Trust from the main commissioner was Hull and East Yorkshire Hospital at 97.13%. There was a positive correlation between deficit size and proportion of income from the commissioner – the more mutually dependent provider and commissioner were the higher the provider's likely deficit, but still with a relatively low r2 of 16.22%.

The funding of CCGs was perhaps as complex as that for providers. Essentially, they received a revenue allocation which was based on the population that they serve, the age of that population, and indicators of deprivation, which was then adjusted for a market forces factor (which estimates the cost differences of delivering care throughout England). This generated a formula for the level of funding the CCG (or previously a PCT) which they should have been getting each year to create an allocation based on a unified weighted population, shown in Figure 4.9.

Figure 4.9 – The Author's CCG allocation calculation methodology

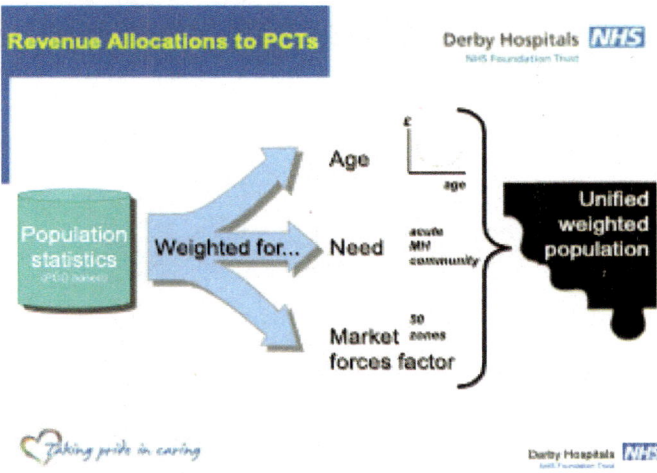

At that point, when growth money was distributed into the English NHS it was done concerning this unified weighted population and the actual allocation. The difference between this proposed allocation and the money the CCGs received was called the CCGs' "distance from the target. Some CCGs got higher allocated growth each year, to move them closer to their calculated allocation, under the funding formula. Other CCGs received less growth in funding, if they received more funding than the allocation methodology suggested they should be getting, as they were above their target allocation.

4.4.5 Financial Performance versus CCG Financial Performance

In addition to whether CCGs were in receipt of their correct funding or not it was then possible for CCGs to be in surplus or deficit. They could be spending, respectively, less or more, than their allocated funding, to generate a surplus or a deficit. The next variable used to model the provider deficit was related to their host CCGs' own surplus/deficit position. As we saw from the last regression, however, the relationships between provider organisations and their commissioners were many and varied. Overall, the CCGs were on plan in terms of their overall finances with an average small surplus of 0.32m. The largest CCG deficit was in North Devon CCG with a total deficit of £120.55m. The largest CCG surplus was £31.83m at Chelsea and Westminster CCG. There was a minimal correlation variable associated with this regression and a very low r2 of 0.3. Therefore, the author re-performed the analysis by only keeping the trusts that had a 50% stake from their main CCG. This left 114 Trusts in the analysis and did produce a positive correlation, but only saw the r2 rise to 0.56%.

Figure 4.10 – Regression 5 – Deficit percentage of Trusts compared to level of CCG deficit.

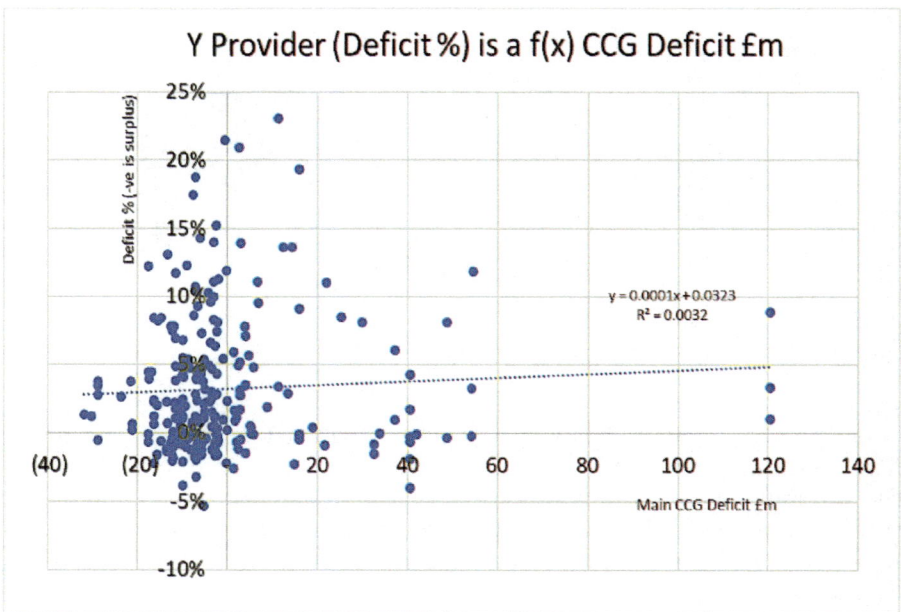

4.4.6 Financial Performance versus CCG Distance from Target

The next variable modelled was associated with CCG distance from the target. Here the mean distance from the target for all CCGs was 0.00%, which should be expected. The maximum amount under target was 5.00% at Manchester CCG. The maximum amount over the target was 30.51% at Chelsea and Westminster CCG. Again, there was a very low correlation coefficient and a low r2 of 0.04%. Also, because of the low interdependencies between some providers and CCGs, the regression was reperformed with only 50% of most interdependent provider Trusts left in this analysis. This only moved the resultant r2 to 0.08%, however.

Figure 4.11 – Regression 6 – Deficit percentage compared to CCG Distance from Target

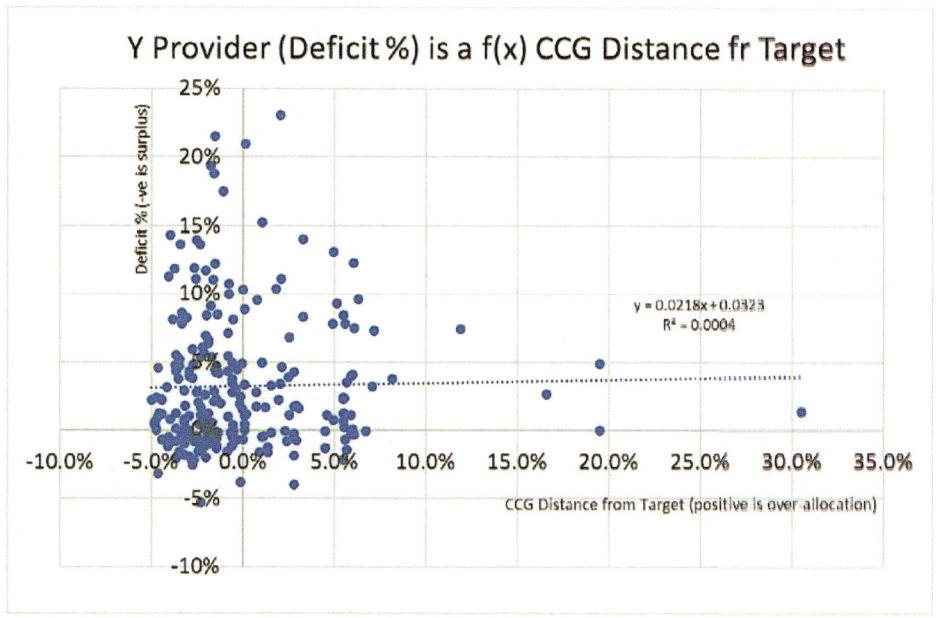

4.4.7 Financial Performance versus Market Forces Factor

The next variable that is modelled looks at the Market Forces Factor. Each provider and CCG has an associated MFF which adjusts the prices they receive for services and the allocations they receive for the commissioning of services. The MFF described by Monitor/NHSE (2013) is:

> The Market Forces Factor (MFF) is an estimate of unavoidable cost

differences between healthcare providers, based on their geographical location. The MFF is used to adjust resource allocations in the NHS in proportion to these cost differences, so that patients are neither advantaged nor disadvantaged by the relative level of unavoidable costs in different parts of the country. (Monitor/NHSE (2013); 2)

The Market Forces Factors for provider organisations vary from 0.93 as a minimum, to 1.20 as a maximum. There is therefore considered to be a 29% difference between the costs of NHS providers within the English NHS based on the geographical location of where the service is offered. The correlation between the overall level of surplus and deficit of providers and their MFFs was weak. There was a correlation in the direction of the higher the MFF the lower the deficit, but again the r2 coefficient is a low 0.29%.

Figure 4.12 – Regression 7 – Deficit percentage compared to Market Forces Factor

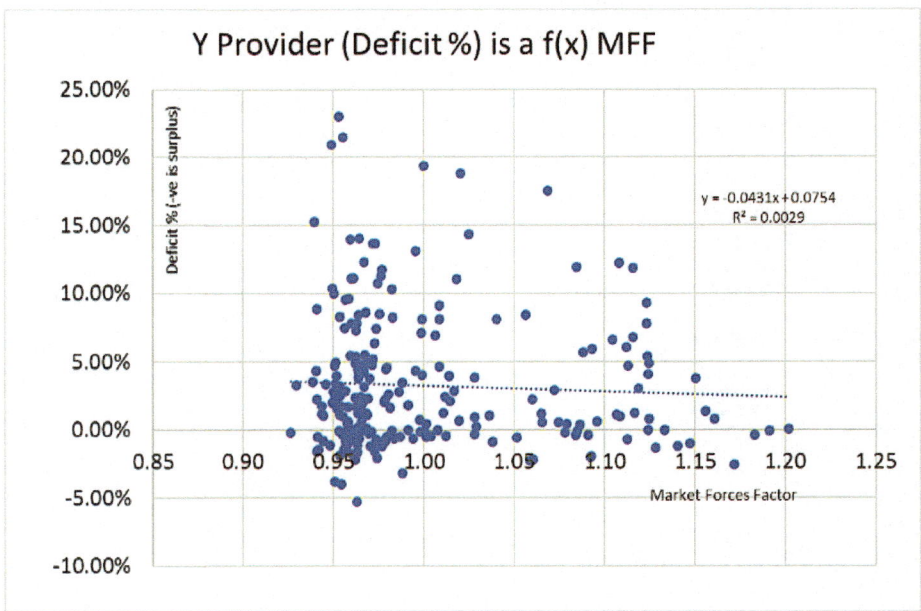

4.4.8 Financial Performance versus NHSE Income

The next variable modelled relates to the proportion of income which the provider received from NHS England for their more specialist and nationally commissioned as opposed to locally commissioned by CCGs. There is a sensible logic to the fact that services are so specialist that they are either planned or commissioned at a national level. The total commissioning spend to providers was spent at an overall ratio of £14.5bn from NHSE for specialist services versus £71.9bn via CCGs in 2016/17.

This ratio between providers was hugely different based on the nature of the services that they delivered. The highest ratio of any provider receiving their income delivered through a specialist commissioning, NHSE route, was 73.7%. Some NHS providers received no income at all from specialist commissioning. The average NHSE income in all providers was 14.5%. Provider deficits were lower based on the proportion of spend that came via the specialist commissioning route and NHSE. However, the r2 associated with the correlation was a relatively low 1.1%.

Figure 4.13 – Regression 8 – Deficit percentage compared to NHSE % income to Trust:

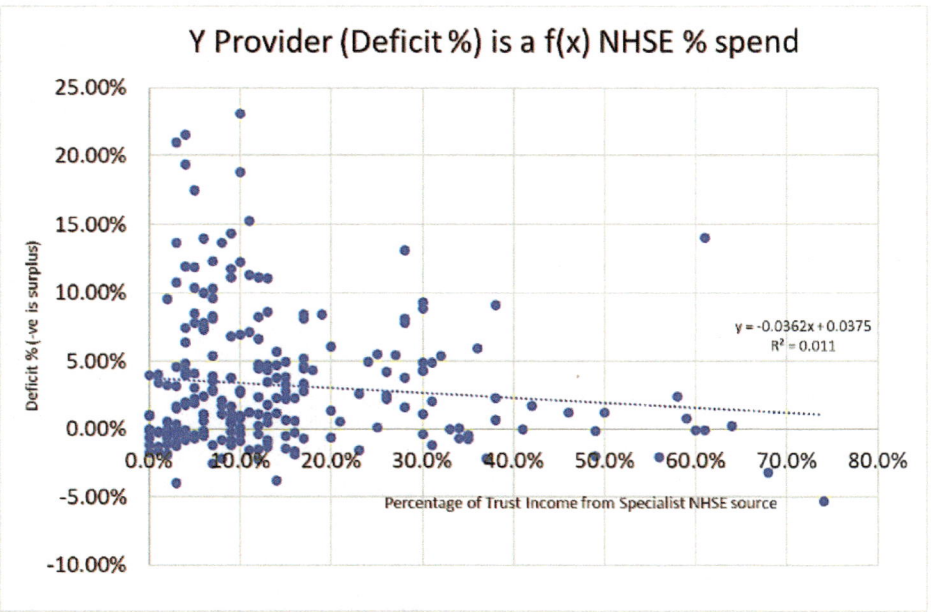

4.4.9 Financial Performance versus PFI Assets

A further significant area of discussion regarding the drivers of deficits in NHS provider organisations has been related to the Private Finance Initiative (PFI). PFI is a funding approach, described by the House of Commons Treasury Committee (2011), which has been used since 1992 to design, build, finance and operate some public sector infrastructure projects, such as hospital building programmes.

This is another one of the live debates in health finance, around how to finance further capital requirements. At the time of writing the English NHS has PFI assets in operation valued at around £11.1bn. There has been a significant skew of assets amongst providers with some having no PFI assets and others having a high concentration.

The highest PFI asset cost in an individual trust is Barts with £1.2bn. The lowest Trust has a PFI asset at only £10m. To see if the deficits were being driven by the concentration of PFI assets costs the correlation has taken place versus PFI Assets as a proportion of trust turnover. There are many Trusts with no PFI assets. The highest PFI asset-based Trust as a proportion of turnover is Barts at 114.1%, and the average PFI as a proportion of turnover for all Trusts is 20.0%. There was a positive correlation with the PFI asset base and a more significant r2 than some of the regressions with 4.83%. It was perhaps likely that PFI is causing deficits, due to average prices funding services and PFI making the cost base of some Trusts more expensive than the average, although not absolutely statistically significantly.

Figure 4.14 – Regression 9 – Deficit percentage compared with PFI Assets

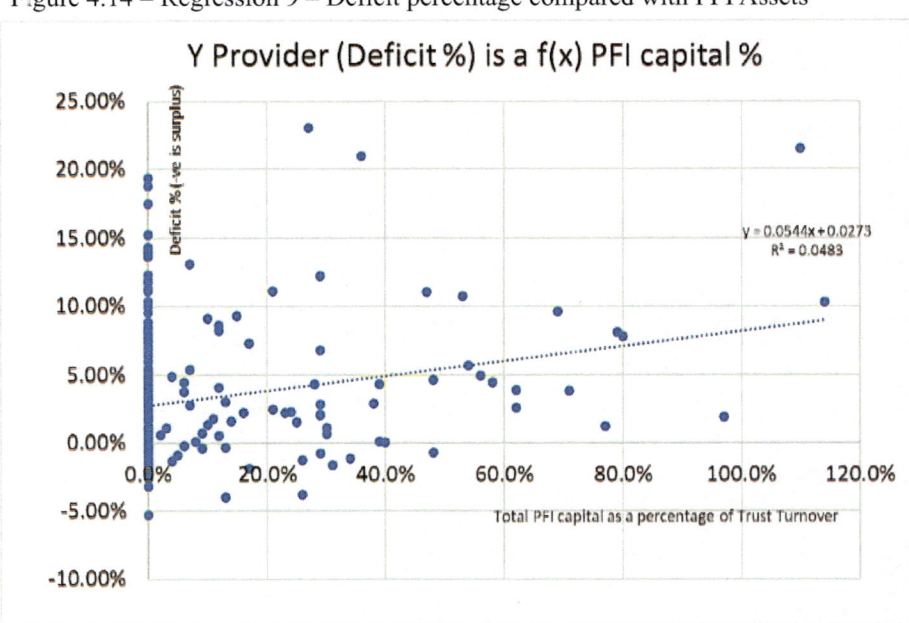

4.4.10 Financial Performance versus Education and Research Income

The next analysis of the potential contributors to healthcare organisation surpluses and deficit is the proportion of income they get from education, training and research. This addresses a narrower subset of non-healthcare-related NHS income than Regression 3, above. Different NHS providers have different degrees of educational and non-commercial clinical trial research activity, which generate alternative funding streams for hospitals and other provider organisations.

The average proportion of income that was derived from education and training and research for NHS organisations is 4.0%. There are several Trusts that derive very little income from this source and the maximum amount of income from this source was a single outlier at 43.8%. This Trust, Tavistock and Portman, is an outlier as a particular specialist Trust. There is no great correlation coefficient from this data and there was a low r2 of 0.29%, which was not improved by removing the Tavistock and Portman outlier.

Figure 4.15 – Regression 10 – Deficit percentage compared with education and research income.

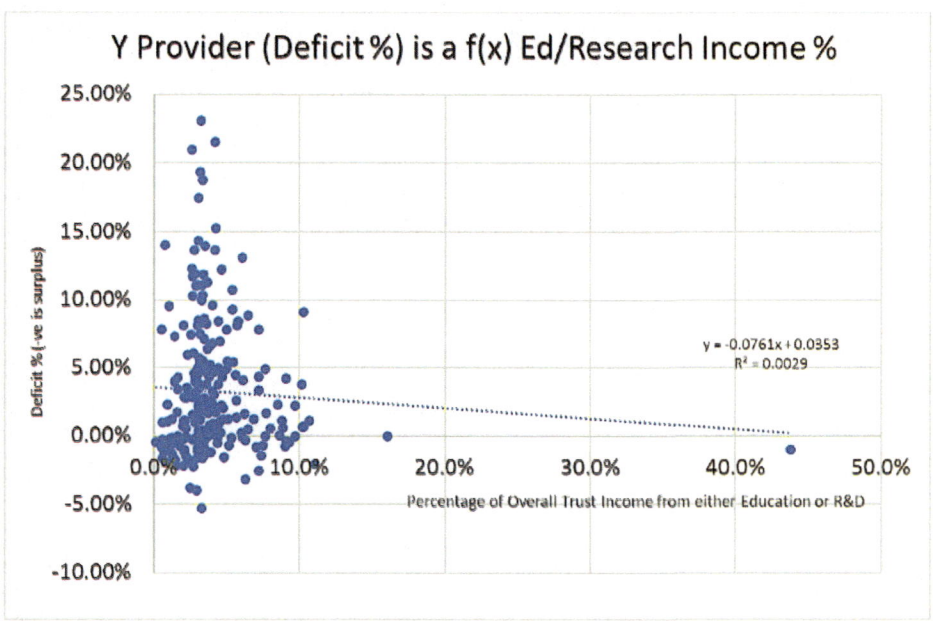

4.4.11 Financial Performance versus CQC Rating and Four-Hour Wait Standard

The next two regression analyses were done at the specific request of an earlier meeting of the HFMA Policy and Research Committee and sought to address if there was any trade-off between quality or performance and financial performance. Put simply: Trusts may be spending more money than the allocation system allowed to achieve a higher Care Quality Commission (CQC) rating or delivering the A&E four-hour standard, resulting in a correlation with deficits. The CQC began its work in April 2009 and replaced the Commission for Social Care Inspection, the Healthcare Commission and the Mental Health Act Commission. The CQC was created by the Health and Social Care Act (HSC Act) 2008. The CQC inspection regime and rating system now grade NHS providers (along with care homes, GP Practices and a number of other health bodies) on a four-point scale; inadequate, requires improvement, good and outstanding (as is the case with Ofsted in schools, and other educational institutions).

Performance targets have been set for the treatment of emergency patients since the 1990s. By 2004, the target stood at, at least 98% of patients attending an A&E department must be seen, treated, and admitted or discharged in under four hours. The target was further moved to 95% of patients within four hours in 2010, because of the coalition's claims that 98% was not clinically justified. These areas are quite highly charged and debated, but the author is disinclined to enter those debates here. For the purposes of this work, the NHS organisation's performance on both the CQC rating and then the Four Hour Wait Performance versus the surplus/deficit measure for 2016/17, was assessed using bivariate regression.

Figure 4.16 – Regression 11 – Deficit percentage compared to Care Quality Commission Rating

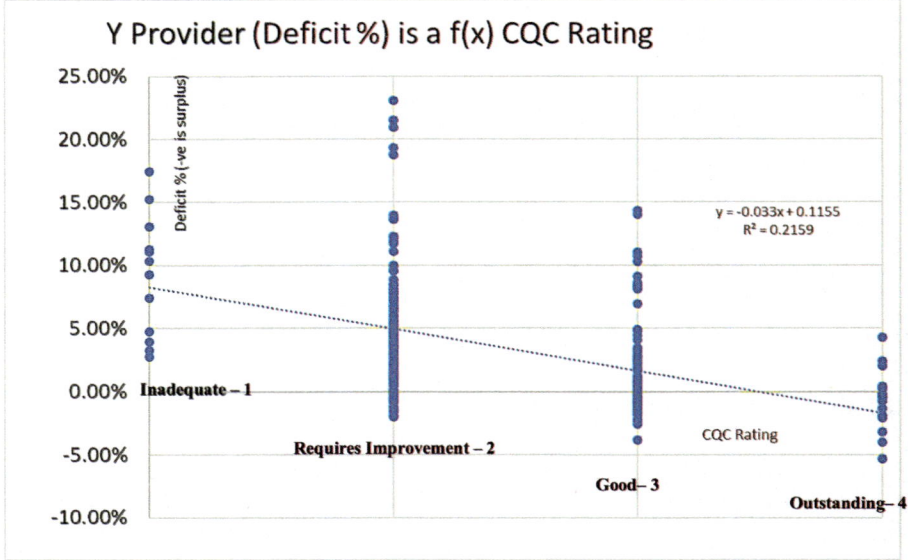

The results of the mapping of provider deficit surplus to the current CQC rating show a reasonably strong negative correlation, with an r2 of 21.59%. In March 2018, there were 12 NHS providers rated Inadequate, 101 rated Required Improvement, 102 rated Good and 15 rated Outstanding. Despite the Policy and Research Committee's view, that chasing a higher quality rating was costing the NHS money (which it could still be) the position is that those with higher ratings (Good and Outstanding) were financially performing better than those that with lower ratings (Inadequate or Requires Improvement). Which way the causality runs in this, and the other elements of the linear regression could be contested, and this was discussed further in the HFMA Policy and Research stakeholder group. Perhaps it is easier to deliver a good and outstanding quality performance in an organisation that isn't financially challenged. What factors drive the level of financial challenge have been contested through the earlier regression work.

The comparison of the hospital's financial performance versus the four-hour standard delivered a relatively similar result. The overall performance for the whole sector against the target was 88.94%. The worst organisation's performance was 72.37%. A few Trusts with Minor Injuries Units or Eye Casualty Units were achieving 100% performance. Again, there was a negative correlation, so the better the organisation were doing against the four-hour standard, the better its financial performance and the lower its deficit. The overall r2 associated with the regression was 19.88%, higher than some of the other analyses.

Figure 4.17 – Regression 12 – Deficit Percentage Compared with Four-Hour Performance

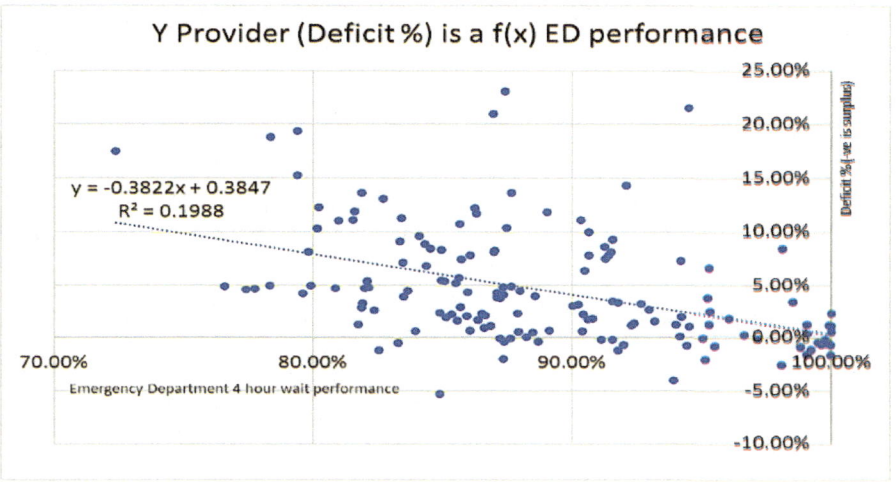

The causes of overall NHS organisation success and failure, not just financial, but on many other measures (clinical, quality, operational and financial) are hugely contested. Some in the Policy and Research Committee (held on 13 February 2018) believed a key indicator would be the continuity of senior management. The role and use of the HFMA Policy and Research Committee is described in section 6.3, below. This continuity of senior management information for each NHS Trust is relatively difficult to collate. Even then, though, there would be contention around whether the period of tenure of the senior management was causing good organisational performance or whether senior managers were more likely to stay because of it, is at issue.

4.4.12 Overall Summary of Financial Performance Regression Work

The approach using regression analysis has shown no correlation with financial performance based on organisational size. Surprisingly, virtually no correlation based on the organisation's relative unit cost efficiency. This was perhaps the most challenging finding if the "could we have a quasi-market with the current funding approach" question were to be answered positively. If there was no correlation between lower unit costs and surpluses, how could the funding mechanism be seen to be running an effective market? The strongest correlation seemingly is in favour of diversifying away from pure NHS treatment and care delivery if financial success is a goal, due to a correlation between these two variables. This could lead towards the conclusion that the core funding to NHS providers was not enough to deliver their services, which may be an intended or unintended consequence of the internal market policy, but perhaps not a stated one.

Table 4.2 – Bivariate Regression Summary Healthcare Organisation Financial Performance

Variable	n	R^2	Conclusion
Deficit £m pre STF	238		Problem re underlying position and non recurrent
Deficit % (Y)	238		
Turnover £M (X1)	238	0.0018	No correlation or effect associated with size
RCI (X2)	238	0.0161	Weak correlation between low RCI and surplus
RC as % Turnover (x3)	234	**0.3446**	Diversification does seem to help
%£ from 1° CCG (x4)	238	**0.1622**	Some correlation, more dependent more deficit
CCG Deficit (x5)	238	0.0032	No correlation between CCG position and Trust
CCG DfT (x6)	238	0.0004	No correlation and CCG/Trust mapping complex
MFF (x7)	238	0.0029	No correlation to MFF
NHSE % (x8)	238	0.011	Weak correlation, more NHSE spend lower deficit
PFI Cap/Turnover (x9)	238	**0.0483**	PFI is a problem, but not strongly correlated
Ed/Research % (x10)	238	0.0029	No correlation to education and research
CQC Rating (x11)	238	**0.2159**	Improving CQC correlates to reducing deficit
ED Performance (x12)	161	**0.1988**	Improving ED correlates to reducing deficit

The correlations between CCG performance and Trust performance are contested, not least because that mapping is so complex, but provider organisations with closer links to one CCG see a correlation with poorer financial performance. MFF and financial performance were not correlated. There was a correlation between Trusts with a higher proportion of income from NHSE for specialist services and surpluses. PFI prevalence did seemingly generate a market distortion that suggests those with a higher PFI base had a correlation with deficits, which was intuitive, due to higher capital and estate costs. Trusts with wider research and education NHS income did see a correlation with surpluses. Higher quality (as measured by CQC rating) and higher performance (as measured by four-hour waiting for standard performance) did not seem to correlated to better financial performance, and the potential causality here between relative financial security and/or more adequate funding and performance is of interest.

4.5 Multivariate Regression of the Healthcare Provider Funding as a Response to the Action Research

An approach to multivariate regression analysis was also undertaken in response to the suggestion from the Policy and Research Committee, which is referred to later in chapters 4 and 5. A member of the committee wondered if regression with all the dependent variables, using a multi-variate regression, might produce a more meaningful result. This would have allowed the significance of each variable to be reviewed, and have would enabled an approach to potentially reviewing the autocorrelation between the independent variables. It was also thought that this may give some significance to some of the variables, such as the MFF, which was not demonstrated by the bivariate regression work performed.

The bivariate models used above, are simple but do not allow an analysis of the contribution of correlation that healthcare organisations' financial performance (Y) is likely to be caused by each one of the explanatory (X) variables. Multivariate regression is defined by Gujarati (1988: 221):

> In the two variable cases, we saw that r2 as defined…measured the goodness of fit of the regression equation: that is, it gives the proportion or percentage of the total variation in the dependent variable Y explained by the (single) explanatory variable X. This notion of r2 can easily be extended to regression models containing more than two variables . . . The quantity that gives this information is known as the multiple coefficient of determination and is denoted by R2; conceptually it is akin to r2.

Sirigari (2020) and Abayomi, Gelman and Levy (2008) both describe the complexity of the different approaches to and the pitfalls of the use of multi-variate regression and how to use diagnostic reports. Sirigari (2020) describes the steps in the development of Multivariate Linear Regression (MLR) Models and the approach to use of data for multi-variate linear regression defining homoscedasticity (where variables have the same finite variance) and heteroscedasticity (where variables have different variances) and multi-collinearity (where the predictive x variables within multivariate regression are themselves linearly dependent). Abayomi, Gelman and Levy (2008) describe three different types of diagnostics that are available for MLR that have helped the author interpret the diagnostic report available within Excel.

The results of the analysis using the multivariate regression, performed in Excel, (with the associated diagnostic report available in Excel) shows:

1. Measured by the Multiple R, which was the correlation coefficient, there was an overall correlation coefficient of 64%. This told us how strong the linear relationship is, between the hospital's financial performance (Y) and all the dependent variables. A value of 100% means a perfect positive relationship and a value of zero means no relationship at all. It is the square root of R squared.

2. R squared. This is R2, the Coefficient of Determination. It indicates how many points fall on the regression line. For example, 80% means that 80% of the variation of y-values around the mean is explained by the x-values. In this case, 40% of the variables fell on the regression line.

3. Adjusted R square. The adjusted R-square adjusts for the number of terms in a model. This tells us that 37% of financial performance was explained by the twelve independent variables, a relatively low coefficient of determination, but showed some significance after adjusting for the number of independent variables. It should be remembered at this point that the highest single r2 was 34.5% in the two-variable model, followed by an r2 of 21.6%, so this relatively low adjusted R2 was to be expected.

4. Observations. The number of observations in the sample, in this case, 238 healthcare organisations.

5. In the second table, the Significance F showed the significance (P-Value) of the whole regression, which was less than 0.05 showing that there was little overall significance to the multi-variate regression analysis.

6. In the third table, the material columns were:

    - Coefficient: which gave the least squares value for the intercept and the individual x variable.

    - P-value: Gave the p-value for the hypothesis test; this column was the significance of each individual variable to the multi-variate regression. As the overall regression P-value, shown by the Significance F value, was significant, this showed which of the individual variables were significant when this value was lower than 0.05.

Based on the overall p-value for the whole multi-variate regression, there was some significance to the multivariate modelling. The analysis gave the overall linear regression equation:

$$y = b + mx.$$

$$y = \text{intercept} + \text{slope} * x.$$

For the twelve variables, the equation would be:

$$y = -0.02 + 0*X1 - 0*X2 + 0.02*X3 - 0.06*X4 + 0*X5 - 0.02*X6 + 0.07*X7 - 0.02*X8$$

$$- 0.03*X9 + 0.14*X10 + 0.02\ X11 - 0.01\ X12$$

Within this equation, however, only turnover (X1), Reference Cost Index (X2), Proportion of Income from main CCG (X4), and CQC rating (X10) have a significant p-value, less than 0.05. The statistical significance for p-values was described by Berry and Sanders (2000: 17): 'Although 0.05 is the widely accepted standard or cut-off level, for statistical significance, researchers may use a criterion that is more liberal (say, the 0.10 level).'

To determine if the less significant variables were invalidating the overall multi-variate regression, the above four variables (X1, X2, X4, and X11), plus Education and Research Income (X10) with a p-value of 0.0969, were also analysed via multivariate regression. The overall Significance F for this second multivariate regression was again significant, with a slightly higher adjusted R2 of 40%. The revised p-values for the five variables, however, left only the Proportion of Income from the main CCG (X4) with a significant p-value of 0.003, all the others were above 0.10. This further result validated the conclusion from the bivariate models that financial performance was not readily explained by the independent variables.

4.6 Conclusions from Discussion on Healthcare Provider Funding Analysis

The approach to both provider-finance and commissioner-finance is complex, and the author would assert that some of the non-practitioner statistical work (such as Cooper et al, 2012) which has been undertaken to try and see whether competition in England has been beneficial or not, does not really get to grips with all of the financial and managerial dynamics in place, and the complexity of the funding environment in operation.

Perhaps, before the overall financial picture for providers worsened from 2015/16 onwards, and before the two instances of the use of the failure regime, via the use of the Trust Special Administrator, there may have been more proponents of the NHS internal market, from within the NHS finance community of practice. Most practitioners now seemed to look at the system, (a) its complexity, (b) potential lack of transparency (the opaque nature of the distressed finance regime, for example), and (c) perverse incentives (which may result in it being difficult for health systems to remain solvent when they reduce the demand for services, for example); and, therefore, struggle to recommend anything other than quite fundamental change. The next Chapter specifically seeks to address and capture those practitioner views further.

CHAPTER 5

FINDINGS — WHAT ARE FINANCE PRACTITIONER'S VIEWS ON THE INTERNAL MARKET?

Utilising the author's insider researcher perspective and access, this chapter looks at the views of the NHS finance profession on NHS finance and the internal market. It reviews some research published in the report HFMA/PwC (2018) "Making Money Work in the Health and Care System". This research undertaken by Price Waterhouse Coopers (PwC – an international accounting, audit and consulting firm) and HFMA sought feedback on answers to whether particular facets of the NHS Finance system could and should be improved, along with qualitative feedback on the existing system. It also tested questions about the pre-pandemic system and whether finance stakeholders agreed with them or not. Furthermore, it allowed gathering a good deal of qualitative feedback, which the author has independently coded, (which was not performed as part of the generation of the actual HFMA/PwC report), that has enabled the capture of further stakeholder opinions on internal market policy. This chapter therefore reviews the extent to which the author's own views, identified in 5.1, below, are in-step with his fellow practitioner colleagues.

This chapter reviews attitudinal research which reviewed practitioner understanding, the scale of impact and the level of support for quasi-market policies with the English NHS, the primary data for which was generated through the HFMA/PwC joint work. This primary data from the HFMA/PwC joint work was made available to the author, via the approval of the rest of the Steering Group, associated with the report, which the author was a member of. The author coded this data, which is later described in this chapter.

5.1 *The Author's Practitioner View on the Internal Market System*

It is worth recounting the work that the author undertook while finance lead for the Derbyshire Sustainability and Transformation Partnership (a forerunner to the Integrated Care Systems, described above) and his previous role as the Director of Finance for Chesterfield Royal Hospital. The author has a relatively unique perspective, as unusually, the hospital in Chesterfield also provides General Practice services in the locality (Royal Primary Care). He is also one of the very few Directors of Finance who have taken on the ICS finance lead role. Despite his relatively unique perspective, the author believes the issues experienced in the local Derbyshire system were echoed around the English NHS and it is valid to recount his own practitioner experience as part of the data on practitioners' views of the internal market. As a finance and management practitioner both in the Derbyshire system and nationally, the author's current role and cumulative NHS experience, continue to shape his views on several critical NHS policy issues. These issues are explored through this thesis, being reflective of the current national English policy debate in the NHS, and they include:

(a) how primary care services work closely with secondary care services in the English NHS,

(b) the nature of the statutory organisations in the health and care system,

(c) the adequacy and effectiveness of the commissioning system

(d) the maturity of the relationships with, and the ability to work jointly with local government

(e) the nature of the oversight role from NHSE and NHSI, and

(f) any residual rationale for the purchaser/provider split.

These issues are discussed in brief in the next section, and from a methodological perspective may be regarded a piece of initial practitioner reflective practice.

Royal Primary Care are the primary care and GP services that are run by Chesterfield Royal NHS Foundation Trust. An increasing number of NHS provider organisations are starting to look at how they work more closely with GP colleagues to integrate care. Consequently, it means Chesterfield has a GP who sits on the Hospital Leadership Team. Integration with the primary care sector to further improve NHS services seems essential to the author, but has not been central to the NHS internal market, since its inception, or, it could be argued, how the NHS was originally founded and brought into national ownership in 1948 (Brown and Payne, 1990).

A reason for the author seeking to be the Director of Finance of the Derbyshire STP was a personal belief that it could have the biggest impact on improving treatment and care for residents, by working more broadly across the health and care system, with system partners, as opposed to solely from working within his own statutory organisation, Chesterfield Royal Hospital. In his previous role at NHSI, the author had been working with NHSE, Treasury, DHSC and London Councils on the devolution agreement on health and care, which sought to form a closer and more formalised working relationship between health and social care in, and for, London. One of the further potential frailties of the NHS internal market has been the lack of formal linkages between health and social care, specifically between the NHS and local government. If these linkages were better, it would enable the system to jointly address socially determined diseases, public health and the broader issues of health and well-being.

The Derbyshire Sustainability and Transformation Partnership (STP) involved the ten main statutory health and care bodies in the county of Derbyshire. There are four provider NHS Foundation Trusts, (two hospitals, one mental health and one community provider); there were four Clinical Commissioning Groups (which have now been through a process to be merged down into one); and two upper-tier local authority bodies (with Derbyshire County Council and Derby City Council, as the two upper tier authorities with responsibility for social care). All ten (seven considering the CCG merger) were actively engaged in the work of the STP. The status of the Derbyshire STP is broadly like the other 42 STPs across England, trying to influence through its non-statutory role in ensuring improvements and care across the geography of the county. The structures which the STP developed were predominately populated from within the current health and care leadership. There was an STP Board with joint accountability to the seven statutory organisations, the two health regulators (NHSE and–NHSI – now a single regulator following the 2022 Act) City and County Health and Wellbeing Boards and the Overview and Scrutiny Committee. This experience amplified the conclusion of the author that the internal market structures in the NHS, and the wider health and social care landscape, were and did make the delivery of integrated and optimal care difficult, which continues to be explored further in this thesis.

In the context of the movement from four CCGs to one more strategic commissioner for Derbyshire, it has already been suggested that the commissioning structure is not quite fit for purpose. A number of areas of the country were changing the scale of the CCGs in the commissioning system to try and ensure they were more effective, impactful and coterminous with the STP/ICS boundary. One telling issue on the adequacy of the commissioning system related to some work which was being undertaken to better understand how patients use the overall services offered across providers. How the data are still held with the four Derbyshire NHS providers and the two local government bodies does and did not easily allow the system to see where there is scope to change and tailor care, based on the current resource consumption of patients across the system. Consequently, a piece of work which is continuing to be developed in Derbyshire is enabling, (a) an understanding of the patient-level resource consumption map across the county, by GP practice and care homes, (b) to enable a plan to integrate and deliver improved care. As a system was and is still very difficult to deliver this work from within the existing statutory structures. This key system requirement, in the author's view, and not being able to deliver it via the pre-existing structures shows the frailty of the commissioning system. This is not unique to Derbyshire and undermines the effectiveness of the commissioning and wider system, in terms of the data it had and has available to it to effectively run a healthcare system. Essentially data for primary care use to shape care services is not and cannot be helped by commissioners in a patient-identifiable way. The provider collaborative in Derbyshire was seeking to perform this care integration analysis to enable a better understanding of the allocative efficiency and triple-value healthcare, which was not possible by commissioning colleagues, in this way.

The maturity of the relationships with and the ability to work jointly with local government in Derbyshire was quite strong in the opinion of the author. There was a track record in developing structures to enable the health and care system to work together well. There was also a good system working to try and ensure there were relatively low numbers of patients unable to leave the hospital due to inadequate provision of care closer to home. One of the "delivery and implementation workstreams" for the Derbyshire STP was the place workstream, managed by the Place Development Board, which sought to try and ensure that there is a common approach to maximise health and wellbeing across the county, by trying to forge a shared plan. The author would contend that the strength of local government engagement through this structure and the historic approach to joint working was relatively good in this region, compared with some of the approaches in the other 42 STP areas. Derbyshire had one of the best national performances relating to Delayed Transfer of Care – a measure of patients waiting to leave the hospital which is sometimes seen as a barometer of the health and local government relationship. Although the non-statutory mechanisms being developed in Derbyshire were reasonable, the author believes a clearer statutory role for local government engagement in the delivery of optimal health and care integration is a key challenge for NHS and local government structures.

The nature of the oversight role from NHSE and NHSI was being challenged by the system to note the need for a coordinated regulatory voice in the system. This was trying to avoid messages from NHSE to the CGG being at odds with messages from NHSI to the four NHS providers. Both NHSE and NHSI were deploying a common regional structure, a change in the approach to oversight in the system. The Derbyshire system volunteered to do some joint work to try and understand how it would begin to operate as an Integrated Care System (ICS) in advance of the 2022 Act.

The statutory organisations in the Derbyshire system were under intense pressure to deliver changes and improvements in care. There was a range of non-statutory structures, attempting to potentially improve, and co-ordinate, the delivery of care which were not reliant on a specification or contracting directive from the old CCG or the emergent strategic commissioner. The providers were equally engaged in trying to deliver changes in service delivery and the precise role of the strategic commissioning and the STP structures, as in other regions, were unclear.

Any residual rationale for the purchaser/provider split was therefore, via the actions of the actors in the system, and the regulators themselves, (despite the statutory need for some of the 'old' structure) were being challenged. There were, in fact, elements of the old structure which were duplicative and inadequate, and there was work underway to try and replace and develop them in a more integrated and locally tailored way, which was heralded in the Long-Term Plan and was confirmed by the Health and Care Act 2022. Although the Health and Care Act (2022) gives a larger role to the integrated care boards, much of the previous separation between providers and commissioners, and their responsibilities remain and have not been formally replaced, which will be returned to in Chapter 7.

5.2 The Impact of the Practitioner Views on NHS Market Policy and HFMA/PwC (2018 Report)

The PwC (2016) report "Redrawing the Health and Social Care Architecture: Exploring the Role of National Bodies in Enabling and Supporting the Delivery of Local Health and Care Services" called for a series of fundamental changes to the way in which the NHS in England was then organised. The PwC (2016) report used a range of polling approaches to research the then views of a wide number of stakeholders on the current NHS structure and concluded:

The need for change came through clearly in our polling of the public and of NHS staff for this report. It suggested that there is:

- widespread confusion over the role of national bodies among NHS staff: a large majority of senior staff in the NHS are not clear on the role of the NHSE (70%) or the DHSC (70%), while only a minority understand the role of NHSI (16%).
- deep frustration with the separation of roles and functions in the health and care system: two in three NHS employees (66%) identified the division between health and social care as a barrier to delivering the vision of local integrated care systems outlined in the "Forward View".
- little clarity about the role of local organisations in improving services: over a fifth of the public hold the Westminster government

responsible for the quality of care in their local hospital or surgery (22%).
- a growing appetite for reform: 71% of NHS staff felt there was a need for change to the current system and only 11% felt that current arrangements were effective. (PwC (2016); 12).

The report had made three specific proposals, therefore, concerning (i) the need to clarify the approach to the national NHS structures and their roles and (ii) the need for a co-ordinating statutory body at the STP/ICS level to co-ordinate local care; and (iii) the need to clarify and integrate elements of the roles of DHSC and DLUHC to help with the national coordination of health and social care. The author had been largely sympathetic to the content of the report and therefore when a further report was proposed, working with HFMA, he was keen to be involved. At the time of the development and production of the 2018 HFMA/PwC Report, there had been some appraisal of the feedback given to the survey involved as part of this work, but the author saw an opportunity to perform further analysis, on the data collected, as part of this thesis.

The Stakeholder Group for "Making the Money Work in the Health and Care System" was chaired by the former Secretary of State for Health, Alan Milburn. It then had three representatives from HFMA, including the author, and three wider NHS finance system stakeholders. Richard Douglas was a former chief of the Government Accounting Service, and the Director of Finance at the DHSC, and was an NHSI Non-Executive Director; Mike Farrar, a former SHA Chief Executive and a former Director General at the DHSC; Anita Charlesworth was Director of Research and Economics at the Health Foundation. The stakeholder group was then supported by the lead from PwC, David Morris, a Partner in their Healthcare Consulting Practice, supported by several further PwC staff.

Following the selection of this project to be incorporated into the thesis, the additional resources which the strand of the research now had at its disposal were considerable and meant the practitioner views associated with the current status of the English NHS finance regime were likely to be considerably more representative. These contributors can be named as ethical consent was gained, and an explanation of the practitioner research undertaken was given to this research group at the time. The Stakeholder Group met monthly between October 2017 and March 2018, to contribute to the research and shape the nature and content of the final Report. The author's role within this Stakeholder Group was multi-faceted. He was simultaneously representing the interests of the HFMA and its Policy and Research Committee and the Trustee. He was also contributing as an existing practitioner in NHS finance, and he was also open about his role; PwC and HFMA were happy and consented to the data from the survey being used as a vehicle for the second research strand of this professional doctorate. The use of this research approach had both benefits and disadvantages. The main benefit surrounded the use of the Stakeholder Group to shape and further influence the author's own opinions on the internal market and NHS finance. This was therefore part of the action research phase of the project, which will be described more fully in the next chapter. As a result of the stakeholder group, the research, therefore, became more collaborative in design and benefitted from further engagement with a number of significant stakeholders in the NHS finance system. There was therefore likely to be a greater impact from the resultant report than if the author had pursued this strand independently, and immediately there would be a product to help with research dissemination. The disadvantage was that the author would not be using the stakeholder questionnaire designed post-pilot, (and couldn't scope the research solely to meet his own research design and purposes), but he believed that this approach could further his research aims and result in actively influencing practice more effectively, and immediately via the HFMA/PwC report that the group produced. However, the work here remains that of the author.

It was also incumbent on the author, as the sole Trustee representative of HFMA, to ensure that the representative views of HFMA members were articulated in the Report. The author, therefore, fed back the status of the joint work with PwC in a series of three HFMA Trustee meetings in October 2017, February 2018 and then finally in May 2018. The Report represents quite an assertive departure for HFMA as it was openly critical of the current NHS finance policy landscape. It also articulated the need for change and documented an important Trustee decision about the extent to which the HFMA would be prepared to be overtly critical of the current NHS finance policy. Also, it was necessary to ensure that the final draft of the Report, if to be jointly branded HFMA and PwC, which it was, did not cause any undue damage to the Association or its membership. All this experience was impactful, in terms of better understanding his own views, the views of practitioners, the views of the Stakeholder Group, and the views of organisations within the NHS structure, to try and generate what was seen to be the view of the professional body representing the NHS finance profession (HFMA).

The questions posed by the research and the responses are shown below. The huge advantage of the PwC work was the administrative infrastructure that helped with capturing all the unpublished data, which the author then had at his disposal for the practitioner view element of this professional doctorate. Had the author needed to capture and administer all the 203 responses to the HFMA/PwC research on practitioner views it would not have been possible to do this as speedily and as accurately or quickly, given the author's full-time job and him fitting in his role as a researcher in his spare time. The research design which the author contributed to as part of the Stakeholder Group specified the survey questions and used the HFMA's membership mailing list to seek responses to the survey. The author could have used his own post-pilot questionnaire using this route but instead took the view that an immediate output to the research in the form of the Report justified the approach to the wider HFMA membership, rather than solely for this professional doctorate research. Although his insider status within HFMA would probably have granted him this access, to pursue his research independently, the utilisation of all HFMAs membership, was more justified for this immediate Report purpose in his view. In addition to the survey, the stakeholder group also commissioned discussions with senior stakeholders in the NHS system, including the Secretary of State for Health, and other senior figures. Overall, the author believed the HFMA/PwC approach was congruent with the action research objective of the thesis.

The questions posed as part of the HFMA/PwC work built on the previous PwC (2016) system architecture report, taking a distinctly more finance-orientated direction. The first four questions of twelve used in the HFMA/PwC practitioner questionnaire sought to understand the nature of the organisations the survey participant worked for (e.g., National Body, provider, commissioner). The second question sought to understand the role undertaken by the participant (e.g., CEO, DoF, Deputy Director of Finance). The third question established the region that each participant worked in. The fourth question sought to understand how the organisation, in which the participant worked, received funding, (e.g., allocation for example to the commissioner, Payments by Results, Block Payment, Capitated Budget, Mix or Other). The next eight questions, HFMA/PwC (2018), were then around attitudes:

    5. The current approach to funding NHS organisations is fit for purpose

    6. The following funding mechanisms encourage organisations to work effectively together

- PbR/tariff
- Block contracts
- Capitated budgets
- CQUIN
- QoF
- Better care fund
- Marginal rate emergency threshold

    7. To what extent do you agree with the following statement - I understand what the financial drivers are for my organisation/role

8. Do you agree with the following statements

   - I expect to be working in some form of integrated care system/organisation in five years.
   - Working in an integrated system will improve patient outcomes/generate value for money.
   - There should be a single budget/I&E for each local health economy (not inclusive of social care and public health).
   - There should be a single budget/Ione for each local health and social care economy not inclusive of public health.
   - There should be a single budget/I&E for each local health, social care and public health economy.
   - Local leaders should be held democratically accountable for the financial performance of health and social care systems.

9. What do you see as the advantages and disadvantages of moving towards a capitation-based system?

10. To what extent do you agree with the following statements about long-term funding?

    - Outcomes would be improved through greater certainty of funding levels over a longer time frame.
    - Unpredictable annual cycles of funding need to be reformed if systems are to be able to engage in sustainable financial planning.
    - National bodies (in particular DHSC) need to maintain access to levers to enable them to influence national priorities.
    - There is a conflict between long-term financial sustainability and short-term efficiency savings.

11. To what extent do you agree with the following statements about outcomes

    - Desired outcome should largely be defined at local level, rather than at national level.
    - Personal patient budgets would be an effective way of driving best use of resources.
    - Linking the way the NHS employees are financially incentivised to decide system outcomes would be an effective way of driving better value.

12. Do you have any additional comments about the way the NHS is funded, and the reforms needed?

The results of the survey therefore were both quantitative and qualitative and their analysis is therefore quite complex, which were used to develop the 2018 Report but were not used as extensively as in the remaining parts of this chapter.

In total, the HFMA/PwC survey received 203 responses perhaps more than possible had the research been pursued solely by the author using his previously intended methodology following on from the pilot study work. The survey was emailed to a total of 900 HFMA members. A wide spread of organisations was represented in the survey responses and roles held by those respondents. The sampling was self-selecting, based on who within the HFMAs membership was willing to participate in the research. It would be difficult to make claims on how representative the survey was of overall finance practitioner opinion on the existing funding system, but with 203 responses there is a considerable depth in the findings of the survey. All the English regions were well represented and there were also responses from members of the national bodies, and some responses from non-English UK HFMA members. There was also a breadth in the funding types, which the research participants had direct experience of, based upon which funding methodology was in place for their organisations, with a relatively even split between allocations (the predominant funding methodology for commissioners), Payment by Results (the predominant funding methodology for hospital providers) and block contracts (the main funding methodology for non-acute providers – community and mental health Trusts).

Question 5. asked the closed question as to whether the research participants felt the current funding system was fit for purpose and this elicited 93 further comments. 152 of the 201 respondents (two survey participants didn't answer this question) did not believe the funding system was fit for purpose, with 20 agreeing it was and 29 unsure. Therefore, of finance practitioners who expressed a preference 88% did not think the existing finance regime was fit for purpose.

Figure – 5.1 - HFMA/PwC practitioner research coding analysis of Q5. "Is funding fit-for-purpose".

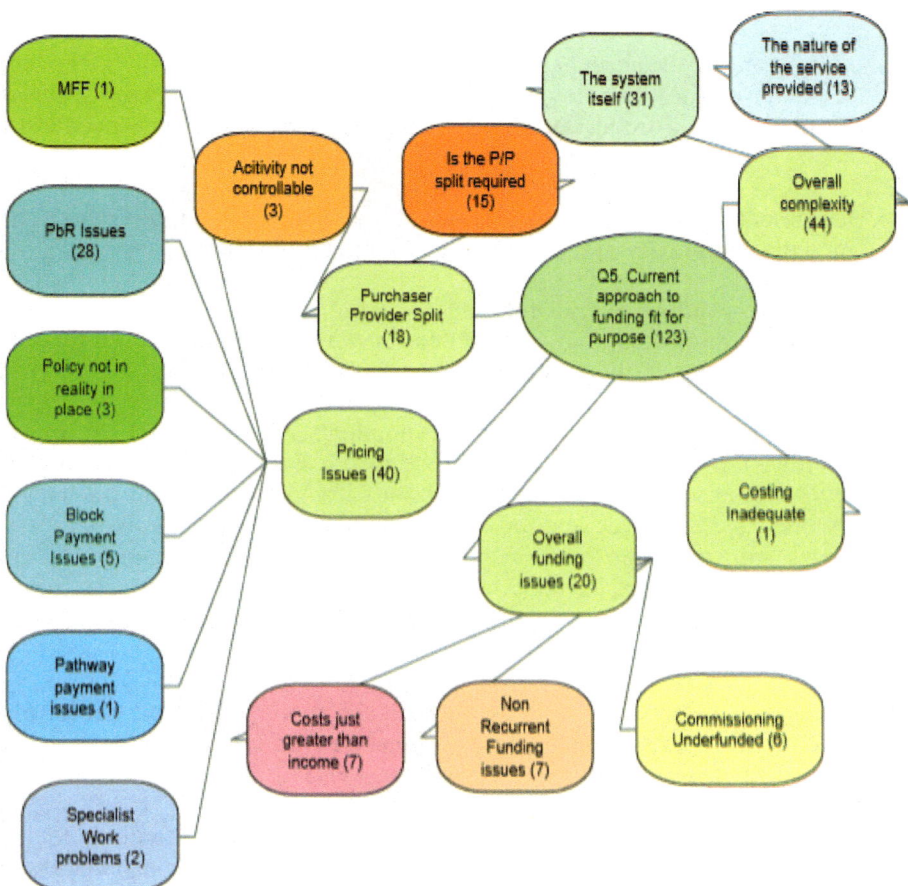

In the context of Question 5, the author split, then coded the written responses into the types listed. This is also illustrated in the coding tree in Figure 5.8, which also shows the rates of responses, associated with each of the answer types, which are:

1. comments on the purchaser/provider split and its adequacy or its requirement, (sub-coded to: if activity cannot be controlled why have the split, and either have a purchaser/provider split or do not)

2. one comment on the adequacy of the costing system to deliver what's needed, (the overall quality of the costing process may be too poor to deliver the required pricing system)

3. comments on the approach to types and kinds of pricing, (MFF is flawed, block payments offer no incentives, PbR is not in place in many systems as it can't be afforded, the activity-based payment system was needed 14 years ago not now)

4. comments on the overall complexity of the system, (both the system itself and the complexity of the services delivered within it)

5. comments on the overall funding available (costs are just greater than income, commissioning isn't funded for the work required, and there is no assessment of the actual funding required overall).

Figure 5.8 shows that out of the 203 respondents, 93 responded as to how and whether they thought the current funding system was "fit for purpose". These 93 responses have generated 123 coded responses, within the 1 to 5 framework listed, above, and in their subsidiary categories. Within the subsidiary categories the main responses were within the category of "the complexity of the system itself" (31), followed by issues related to "Payments by Results" (28), followed by responses coded to the "purchaser/provider split required" category (15).

Regarding the responses on the system itself: there was not a uniformly negative set of responses, but on their coded review a summary position might be given from within this one individual response:

> Tariff works as designed to promote the flow of funding to the 'frontline' of acute and general hospital services at a time of increased availability of funds and a need to increase activity (i.e., 14 years ago). This is not the current state of the health system, but whilst the provisions of and demands on the service have moved on, funding systems have not. (HFMA/PwC Unpublished research, research respondent: 15/02/18 4:20PM ID: 73855111)

The Payments by Results (PbR) answers are somewhat more technical and then describe the required behaviours and other issues in the system, in their response types. The majority noted a need to move our funding approach to match the more recent challenges of the English NHS:

> It's interesting to note we can clearly articulate the policy goals of the 'PbR-era'. I'm not sure we can be as clear about the policy goals of today and, therefore, judge where and in what circumstances particular payment mechanisms are or aren't working. Also, we should not assume that other payment mechanisms don't come with different but equally significant risks. (HFMA/PwC Unpublished research, research respondent: 23/02/18 5:20PM ID: 74643163)

All fifteen responses which used a reference to the purchaser/provider split in response to the funding mechanism being fit for purpose were negative. A typical answer in this coded type was:

> The NHS is currently in flux. We are trying to move away from a purchaser / provider split in some areas without this being legally possible. This leads to complicated systems which are confusing for the general public and the people that work in the NHS. Either get rid of the split or keep it, don't try to do both. (HFMA/PwC Unpublished research, research respondent: 15/02/18 11:12AM ID: 73846614)

Finance qualitative data, therefore, supported the overall negative view on whether the pre-pandemic regime was fit for purpose with specific concerns on the internal market, Payment by Results and the wider payment system. Question 6 reviewed more specifically which elements of the funding mechanism were seen to work better than others. None of the funding mechanisms received majority support, as a route to encouraging organisations to work together. If we had a thriving internal market, to what extent we would need to be encouraging organisations to work together or not, is at issue. The author would claim that the "ship has sailed" on this internal market idea, and the current views within the Stakeholder Group itself, largely supported by the finance practitioner research, and the more recent policy initiatives such as forming Sustainability and Transformation Partnerships, provided evidence of a need to change policy and our approach to running the English health and care services.

Table – 5.1 – HFMA/PwC research on which funding mechanisms help organisations work together.

6. Do you agree that the following funding mechanisms encourage organisations to work together effectively?	Agree	Disagree	Unsure	Response Total
PbR/tariff	21.1% (42)	66.3% (132)	12.6% (25)	199
Block contracts	25.1% (49)	54.9% (107)	20.0% (39)	195
Capitated budgets	46.4% (91)	12.8% (25)	40.8% (80)	196
CQUIN	31.6% (62)	46.9% (92)	21.4% (42)	196
Quality and Outcomes Framework	12.1% (23)	36.8% (70)	51.1% (97)	190
Better Care Fund	24.9% (48)	36.8% (71)	38.3% (74)	193
Marginal Rate Emergency Threshold	6.6% (13)	59.9% (118)	33.5% (66)	197

The payment system for episodic care, Payments by Results, received 21% approval, in keeping with the qualitative comments in Question 5. Block contracts, where the payment is made irrespective of the level of activity performed fared slightly better at 25%. Capitated budgets, which were largely the funding mechanism for CCGs got a higher 47%. CQUIN, (Commissioning for Quality and Innovation) which was an additional payment representing circa 2% of tariff income to providers, which was linked to the performance against particular quality targets got 32% support. QOF (the quality and outcomes framework) which was and is a payment made to GPs for achieving particular quality measures received 12% support. The Better Care Fund, which was a required allocation from CCGs to local government to enable the appropriate social care packages to ensure that care is available outside hospitals received 25% support.

The lowest approval (6.6%) was received by the Marginal rate emergency threshold. This was an adjustment made to the Payments by Results system ten years ago which saw the reimbursement for non-elective or emergency work remunerated beyond a baseline of activity reimbursed at a marginal rate (once 30%, then changed to 70%) which tried to ensure the hospital sector was incentivised to try and take greater ownership of changing the shape of unscheduled care treatment via better outreach and thus delivering care in a less episodic way. The variants to the payment system make it, and their potential correction and change complex, notwithstanding the fact there is a lack of approval for many elements of the approach to the English NHS finance system.

Question 7 sought to establish whether practitioners understand the financial drivers for their own organisations. The majority do, despite the complexity reported previously. Also, it is important to note the further responses, which are described, in the subsequent qualitative coded research about practitioner views on the need for change.

Table – 5.2 - HFMA/PwC research do you understand the financial drivers for your organisation

	7. To what extent do you agree with the following statement? I understand what the financial drivers are for my organisation/role.		Response Percent	Response Total
1	Agree		91.50%	183
2	Disagree		3.50%	7
3	Unsure		5.00%	10

Question 8 looked at stakeholder views associated with changes to move away from the internal market. Over 80% of respondents agreed or strongly agreed that they would be working in some sort of integrated system within five years. Over 70% then either agreed or strongly agreed that these changes would improve patient outcomes and value for money. Over 78% of respondents either agreed or strongly agreed that a move towards a fuller integrated health and social care and public health budget would be best, compared with narrower integration definitions. Over half of the respondents believed that local leaders should be held democratically accountable for the financial performance of the local health and care system. This is a significant result in the context of a group of practitioners, most of whom have only ever worked within the structures that form the internal market.

Table – 5.3 - HFMA/PwC research on a move away from the market to integrated care

9. Do you agree with the following statements?

	Strongly agree	Agree	Neutral	Disagree	Strongly disagree	Response Total
I expect to be working in some form of integrated care system/organisation in five years' time	29.0% (58)	51.5% (103)	11.5% (23)	5.0% (10)	3.0% (6)	200
Working in an integrated care system will improve patient outcomes/generate value for money	20.7% (41)	50.5% (100)	23.2% (46)	5.1% (10)	0.5% (1)	198
There should be a single budget/I&E for each local health economy (not inclusive of social care and public health)	11.5% (23)	30.5% (61)	25.0% (50)	28.0% (56)	5.0% (10)	200
There should be a single budget/I&E for each local health and social care economy (not inclusive of public health)	13.6% (27)	33.2% (66)	24.1% (48)	25.1% (50)	4.0% (8)	199
There should be a single budget/I&E for each local health, social care and public health economy	38.6% (76)	39.1% (77)	9.1% (18)	11.2% (22)	2.0% (4)	197
Local leaders should be held democratically accountable for the financial performance of health and social care systems	19.9% (39)	36.2% (71)	19.9% (39)	17.3% (34)	6.6% (13)	196
					answered	200
					skipped	3

Question 9 sought qualitative opinion on the advantages and advantages of a capitation-based system of funding, which again the author has attempted to code into key themes, as shown in Figure 5.9. There were 137 responses related to capitation-based systems, which were coded into 165 themes, which were split from 81 advantages to 84 disadvantages. Essentially, a move to a capitation-based system could be seen as a movement away from the reimbursement for the activity that has been related to Payments by Results. It could either be seen as the allocation to a new ICS without the purchaser/provider split, or a new contract between purchasers and providers. In the advantages section the three highest coded categories were: could reduce the bureaucracy associated with the current mechanisms in the internal market (23); could promote partnership working across systems (21) and could remove the need for the purchaser-provider split (10). In the disadvantages section: there were a number of examples given of new risks and uncertainties that could be introduced via the new system (36); along with improved management skills that would be required with such a change (8); the required changes in attitudes that would be required with such a change (7); and the potential disadvantages associated with another large scale change in the NHS and the disruption that might cause (7).

Figure – 5.2 – HFMA/PwC research coding on "advantages and disadvantages of capitation-based system"

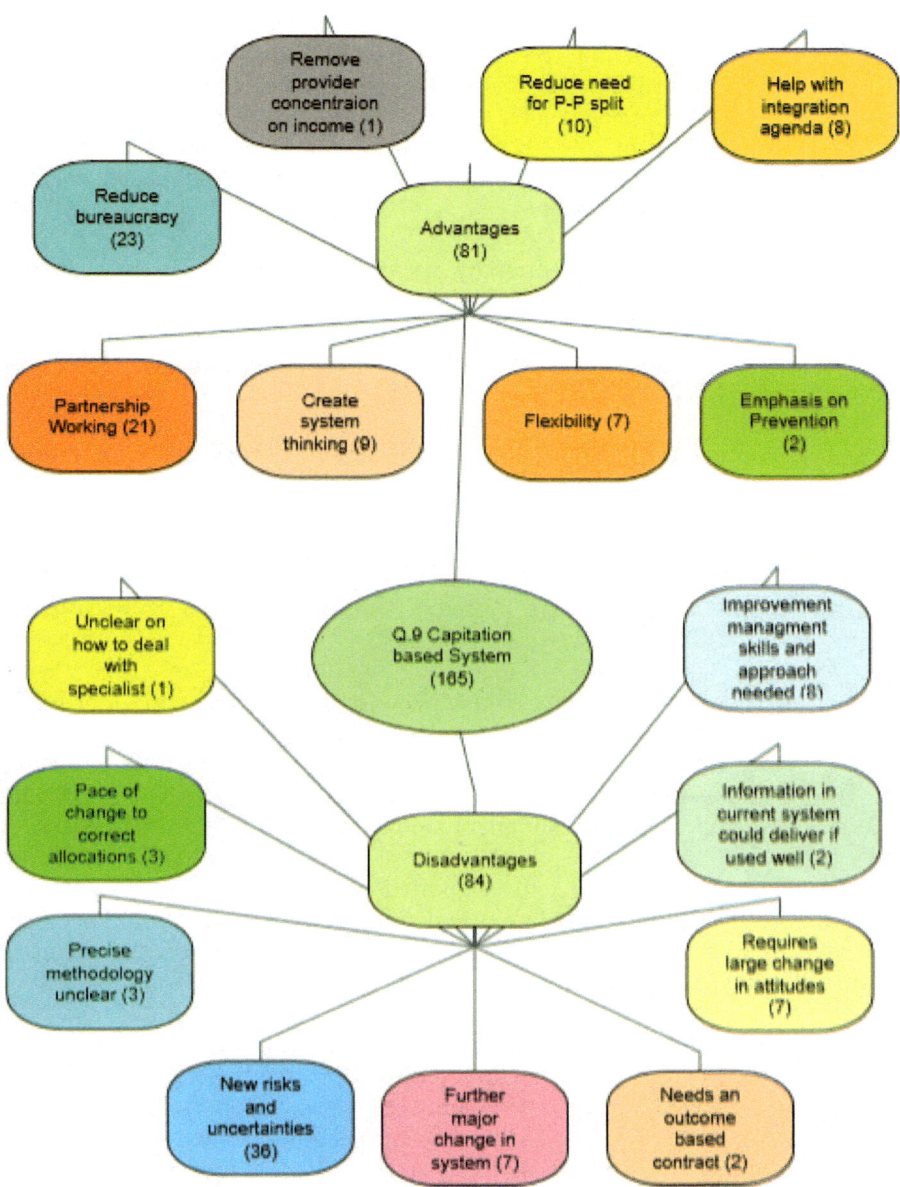

Of the verbatim comments in each of these three subcategories associated with advantages, some of the most representative and or significant include those cited below. All the advantages comments tended towards the need for a radical overhaul of the current financial system in the English NHS, which the move towards a different funding system may necessitate. There was a different emphasis in some of the responses which have moved towards a need for a removal of the purchaser/provider split, including the need to integrate into a new organisational form, after the removal of the split; versus those who have answered from the perspective of the need to modify the extant mechanisms with the current market system:

> Relating to the bureaucracy associated with the current system: - Simpler system, which is easier to understand, more transparent and reduced time and burden of the current complex system. (HFMA/PwC Unpublished research, research respondent: 05/03/18 5:50PM ID: 75742803)

> Relating to the approach to partnership working: - Can remove cost and organisational-centric behaviours of competitive system. System transformation is more effective if system wide. Patient experience/outcomes more likely to be the focus of prioritisation. Removes arbitrary organisational barriers to change. (HFMA/PwC Unpublished research, research respondent: 05/03/18 5:50PM ID: 75742803)

> Relating to the removal of the need for the purchaser provider split: - The current fractured commissioning approach following the Lansley reforms with no-one holding the ring is a disaster. The difficulty lies in STP not being accountable organisations. (HFMA/PwC Unpublished research, research respondent: 06/03/18 11:44AM ID: 75837159)

The disadvantages of the move to a capitated system mainly relate to a move to a new not fully described set of risks and uncertainties, which would need and still need to be addressed. In the specific area of new risks and uncertainties, some of the answers included:

> don't think we (I) fully understand what any of these terms really mean. CCGs receive a capitated budget already, simply moving the risk down the chain does not necessarily solve anything, and creates many risks and grey areas of responsibility, which we will spend much effort trying to manage. (HFMA/PwC Unpublished research, research respondent: 15/02/18 11:49AM ID: 73849363)

> Any capitation-based system will need to work out how to incorporate the priority setting and decision-making bases into their planning processes. There is a strong argument too for greater use of health economics to support the identification of the most cost-effective solutions, but there remains a gap in local democratic accountability for the inherent judgements or decisions. The need to mobilise any preferred solutions might be delayed without pre-existing price, contractual terms and business rules etc. A further disadvantage may also result due to a move from standard cost/price with the potential divergence in levels of efficiency and productivity across providers without a continued cost and efficiency benchmarking process. (HFMA/PwC Unpublished research, research respondent: 15/02/18 4:20PM ID: 73855111)

> in the context of an underfunded NHS at the macro level, capitation potentially leaves providers even more exposed to unfunded pressures of rising demand, how do you resolve the allocation of funds across a multi-provider system, potential to lose sight of service and patient-level costs if currencies are obsolete, sparsely populated areas may lose out as they will by nature be more costly to deliver to. (HFMA/PwC Unpublished research, research respondent: 01/03/18 5:07PM ID: 73846214)

The other three main themes in the coded responses also reveal issues associated with the risks of change. These relate to improved management skills, changes in attitudes that are required and the inherent risks of any further changes:

> Will need significant changes in methods of planning, prioritisation, decision-making. Represents another major change/upheaval for organisations, when stability is needed. Will need a major upshift in scale and quality of planning/management skills. If capitation budgets not set at the right level then just outsources misery. (HFMA/PwC Unpublished research, research respondent: 15/02/18 4:57PM ID: 73882231)

> The disadvantage is that the current system discourages this, and behaviours and relationships are so embedded that implementing this will require a sea change in the attitude, approach and work of many health finance professionals that will be difficult. Clear accountability is key but is not so transparent in a capitation system. (HFMA/PwC Unpublished research, research respondent: 15/02/18 11:19AM ID: 73845719)

Getting there will be hard – lots of vested interests (CSUs, CCGs etc), plus analytical systems not yet of the quality we see in the USA. It will take time. And would be easier if we had a bit of time in the parliamentary calendar to make a few changes to current system. (HFMA/PwC Unpublished research, research respondent: 05/03/18 3:15PM ID: 75728184)

The Long-Term Funding issues are addressed in Question 10, which suggests relatively strong agreement around the need for a more medium-term planning approach. This result is unsurprising and intuitive, at the moment, as the NHS budget continues to be subject to an annual review process which can impede medium and long-term financial planning. In question 10, the result of that is of particular interest to the author is the answer on the need for a national intervention, with 66% of respondents believing in DHSC needs to maintain access to levers to enable change. The author increasingly believes changes to the NHS and social care can only be enabled sustainably at a local level, which is a key tension in the current system and its architecture.

Table 5.4 – HFMA/PwC research on statements about long term funding

10. Do you agree with the following statements about long-term funding?	Agree	Disagree	Neutral	Response Total
Outcomes would be improved through greater certainty of funding levels over a longer timeframe	77.3% (150)	10.8% (21)	11.9% (23)	194
Unpredictable annual cycles of funding need to be reformed if systems are to be able to engage in sustainable financial planning	91.2% (177)	2.6% (5)	6.2% (12)	194
National bodies (and in particular DHSC) need to maintain access to levers that enable them to influence national priorities	66.0% (128)	9.3% (18)	24.7% (48)	194
There is conflict between long term financial sustainability and short-term efficiency savings	83.2% (159)	8.4% (16)	8.4% (16)	191
			Answered	194

Question 11 sought to further understand practitioner views on where the required outcomes for the system were defined, the support for personal patient budgets and the extent to which practitioners believe linking the way NHS employees were remunerated to system outcomes would improve delivery. There was an even split in the decision around whether the required outcomes should be described at a local as opposed to the national level, with a small majority in favour of setting outcomes at a local level, agreeing with the author's own view.

Table 5.5 – HFMA/PwC practitioner research on statements about outcomes

11. To what extent do you agree with the following statements about outcomes?				
	Agree	Disagree	Neutral	Response Total
Desired outcomes should largely be defined at the local level, rather than at a national level	37.8% (73)	32.6% (63)	29.5% (57)	193
Personal patient budgets would be an effective way of driving best use of resources	12.4% (24)	56.7% (110)	30.9% (60)	194
Linking the way that NHS employees are financially incentivised to desired system outcomes would be an effective way of driving better value	27.1% (52)	47.9% (92)	25.0% (48)	192
			answered	194
			skipped	9

There was little support for the concept of assigning personal patient budgets, with only 12.4% in favour of their use. The majority of respondents disagreed with the idea of linking the way NHS employees are financially incentivised to desired system outcomes, with only 27.1% in favour. There were 48 additional comments in response to the statements on outcomes. These were coded to 74 different themes with 29 on national outcome definition, 28 on how individual NHS employees are financially incentivised, and 19 on personal health budgets.

The majority of responses on outcomes support the view that outcomes should be defined nationally to avoid any sort of postcode lottery (11) are shown in Figure 5.2. Some responses supported the need to define outcomes both nationally and locally (7), with others requiring further definitional work on outcomes before they could be supported (4).

> I believe outcomes should be defined at a national level with the methods of delivery determined at a local level. Outcomes should be clear outcome measures (rather than output measures), with success based on delivering outcomes (health or determinants of health), not outputs (activity). (HFMA/PwC Unpublished research, research respondent: 15/02/18 4:20PM ID: 73855111)

Of the 19 comments on personal health budgets, there were 16 negative comments compared with 4 positive comments. The comments included:

> Personal health budgets would not drive better use of resources. Giving each citizen a budget would effectively destroy the founding principle of the NHS and also create a massive administrative burden. Individuals should be empowered to self-care and self-

> manage however not everyone is capable of or wants to make the best decision or use public funds in the best way. (HFMA/PwC Unpublished research, research respondent: 05/03/18 6:34PM ID: 75747271)

> Personal budgets would be the ideal way, but much investment needs to be done to transform the way the NHS works and records activity of people funded this way. Signing a budget off is one thing. Tracing how that money has been spent in organisations requires a shift in operating. (HFMA/PwC Unpublished research, research respondent: 05/03/18 3:18PM ID: 75728096)

The majority of the responses, 16 compared to 9, believed that trying to incentivise individuals financially to achieve system outcomes may not be helpful, with responses ranging from:

> It would hold people to account for making certain decisions currently the NHS doesn't do this (HFMA/PwC Unpublished research, research respondent: 23/02/18 10:30PM ID: 74670134); to.

> Local leaders cannot be held accountable for national decisions and health and social care are so complex that holding an individual leader accountable for population's individual decisions on lifestyle choices and the financial impact of those individual choices seems unacceptable. Additionally, it is already difficult enough to get good public sector leaders at the salaries on–offer - do we really want to completely drive everyone out? (HFMA/PwC Unpublished research, research respondent: 08/03/18 8:40AM ID: 76077256)

Lastly the survey sought practitioner additional comments on the way the NHS is funded, and the reforms needed, which have then also been coded in terms of their responses. The most popular response related to the area coded to "national system management" issues. The author has split these into the six overall coded themes, shown in Figure 5.3. The largest number of responses related to the need to ensure that changes to the approach to the way the system itself is managed should take place nationally.

> It desperately needs the internal market to be abolished, for the number of organisations to be reduced, and for us all to work for one NHS, rather than the current system which encourages the pursuit of individual organisation objectives at the expense of the greater system. (HFMA/PwC Unpublished research, research respondent: 15/02/18 11:42AM ID: 738500956)

Figure 5.3 - HFMA/PwC practitioner research coding analysis of Q11 "outcomes"

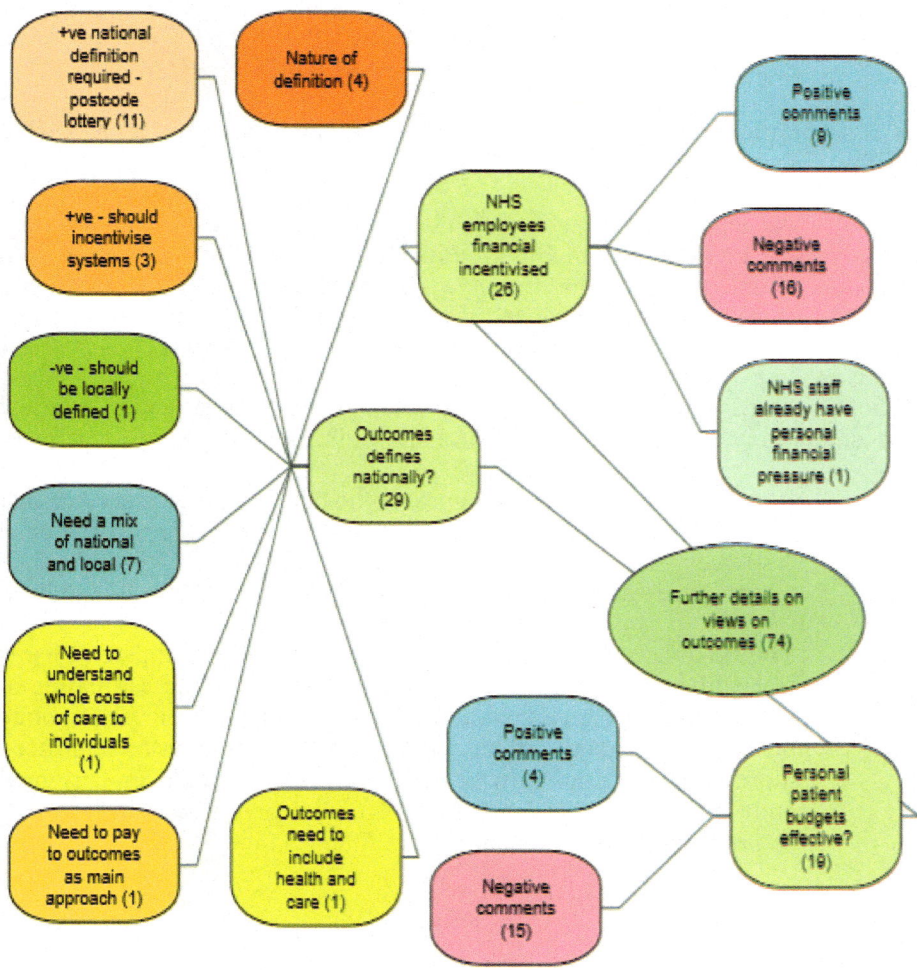

The framing of questions feels biased towards a specific set of answers that we feel major changes are the way forward. I worked in the NHS when there were only directly managed units and waiting times for example were horrendous. (HFMA/PwC Unpublished research, research respondent: 15/02/18 6:17PM ID: 73891571)

Need one system, nationwide. Mandate everything. The simplest way would be a centrally controlled fund, paid to a single body on a capitated basis. Cut out all of the commissioning levels. Mandate the

> type and level of care to be provided nationally, no postcode lottery. Mandate all systems, so that we do not have hundreds of variations all trying to reinvent the wheel. (HFMA/PwC Unpublished research, research respondent: 08/03/18 7:58AM ID: 75352916)

The second-highest series of responses related to the overall funding available within the system.

> As noted, the total funds in are not enough at the moment and the commitment to EU GDP average investment % has not been maintained. Without this any changes to internal financing structure is really "deckchairs on the Titanic time". (HFMA/PwC Unpublished research, research respondent: 15/02/18 11:19AM ID: 73845719)

The next two joint highest response rates relate to the wider political considerations around the system and the definition of the system itself.

> We need an open conversation with the public about the service that should be provided and what we can provide within the non-financial resources that we have available. (HFMA/PwC Unpublished research, research respondent: 15/02/18 11:17AM ID: 73845698)

> The WHO has previously identified (?2008) the social determinants of health and this goes wider than the level of healthcare funding or provision in any given country. It is shown that wider social policy directly or indirectly affects health and this too must be addressed more explicitly. Looking at health funding in isolation is short-sighted and inadequate. (HFMA/PwC Unpublished research, research respondent: 15/02/18 4:20PM ID: 73855111)

Figure 5.4 - HFMA/PwC research coding analysis "The NHS is funded and the reforms needed".

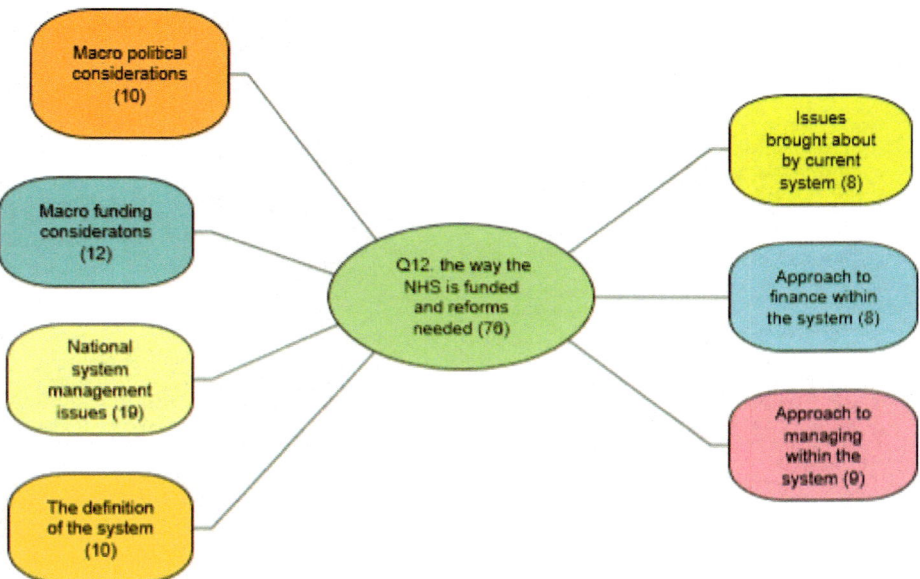

Within the HFMA/PwC work, there is a rich body of qualitative data that has enabled the author to further validate the overall findings and recommendations in the report. The report's findings are summarised in Figure 5.4 and in the bullet list below:

- finance practitioners did not think the current system was fit for purpose.
- they believed largely that the purchaser/provider split had passed its sell-by date.
- the components of the current funding system were not supported (MFF, PbR, block contracts).
- the system was seen as over-complex, and a longer-term funding settlement is needed.
- there was a belief that the overall level of funding was inadequate, but it is hard to tell, due to the complexity and the bureaucratic nature of the existing system.
- the old system needed replacing with something that is fitter for the challenges ahead around more integrated care with social care for the growing elderly population.
- there was nervousness about the new model to be adopted and the risks and uncertainties associated with that; and nervousness about

the risks associated with a further major change to the system or the funding approach within it.

Figure 5.5 - Summary Schematic of the HFMA/PwC report findings

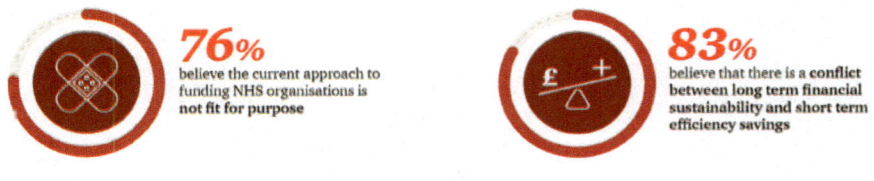

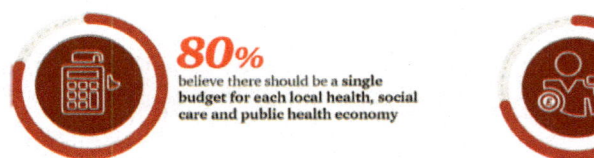

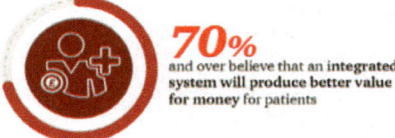

The third aim of the research was specifically to try and influence policy by making a case for change. The HFMA/PwC Reports contents have been discussed at a number of subsequent conferences. The author has spoken alongside Alan Milburn at an NHS provider conference and as part of this process, further stakeholder views were gathered on the Report's contents. In summary, the HFMA/PwC (2018) Report concluded:

> Current funding flows do not support the move towards place-based care and worse still are acting as a significant blocker to system change. This is not at all surprising given their design some 15 years ago was linked to policy objectives aimed at: bringing down waiting lists by incentivising greater throughput from providers; bringing new capacity into the market from private providers and encouraging competition.
>
> The funding mechanisms enabling these policy objectives have yet to be restructured to match the more recent emerging preference for place-based integrated care and cooperation among organisations within systems. In many parts of the country, commissioners are attempting to move away from national payment mechanisms towards various forms of 'aligned incentive' or block contracting in an attempt to share risks and foreshadow place-based work. But this brings its

own risks, not all of which are yet understood, and makes the current position even more confusing and potentially misaligned. Without realigning the way money flows through the system, there is a high risk that the new objectives will not be successfully implemented, and the system transformation will be unable to achieve its goals.

It is a welcome the development that new models of care focussed on delivering more outcomes and value-based care are now starting to emerge. Other countries – often with very different health systems – are following a similar pattern. So, strategically, England's system seems to be moving in the right direction. But the way the NHS financial system currently works is simply not aligned with place – and outcome-based care. Today the care system and the way that money moves around it is in a messy no man's land with a chaotic and bewildering array of financial mechanisms in place. (HFMA/PwC (2018); 4)

The next chapter reviews the wider role of finance practitioners in influencing public policy in the English NHS, and how the author has continued to try and exert that influence, to try and move away from the "messy no man's land with a chaotic and bewildering array of financial mechanisms".

CHAPTER 6

FINDINGS - HOW DO FINANCE PRACTITIONERS INFLUENCE POLICY?

This chapter describes the development and responses to the growing realisation that the nature of the English NHS finance regime and the internal market need to change. Key to this is the emergence of first plans, then structures, initially called Sustainability and Transformation Plans, then Sustainability and Transformation Partnerships, and the idea of the health and care constituent organisations working more closely together beyond the internal market structure. The informal, senior-level feedback on the HFMA/PwC report was that there was a full awareness that there was a need for a legislative change in the English NHS statutory framework, but not then the legislative time or parliamentary majority to effect that change. This has now been addressed and is a central aim of the Health and Care Act 2022. This chapter also describes the action research that the author has undertaken, both in his role within the Policy and Research Committee of the HFMA and for the Public Policy and Reform Faculty Board at CIPFA.

As described in Section 3.8, this chapter therefore describes the action research phase of the thesis which sought to provide the results of the first two research objectives, back to practitioners, operating within the NHS quasi-market area: extending both their and the author's understanding of these policies and their impacts, through the HFMA Policy and Research Committee. This approach is documented below and in Appendices 7 to 17.

6.1 The Role of Evidence in the Development of Public Policy

At the start of this professional doctorate process, the author was keen to understand the notion of evidence-based policy or management in the context of the English NHS. The more that the author has worked on this thesis the more he has become interested in not only the nature of the English NHS system, and finances, but also in the complex map of how policy is shaped and influenced with and by the English NHS.

The English NHS landscape is scattered with numerous organisations with different roles and degrees of power in the system. If one were to try and influence policy, it would be difficult to know where to start. The author has attempted to map out the different environments in which health policy could be developed. Although not comprehensive, it outlines the arenas where policy may be influenced. If one managed to generate some evidence on how the future of the English NHS finances should be structured – even if this were uncontested, which is somewhat difficult to imagine in social science and public policy – where would a practitioner/researcher take the evidence to try and effect a positive change to the system? Figure 6.1 gives some credence to the claims that have been made to establish a Royal Commission to discuss a long-term funding settlement for the NHS. There have been several suggestions to develop a Royal Commission (relatively recently by the Centre for Policy Studies - A Royal Commission on the NHS: The Remit (2018)) to review how the NHS is funded, perhaps with a non-political body making a recommendation on funding levels, akin to the neutrality of the Bank of England on interest rate setting. It may also make sense to extend that Commissions work to how we should organise the system.

Figure 6.1 – An Original Summary Schematic of the Complex Map of How NHS Policy is Shaped

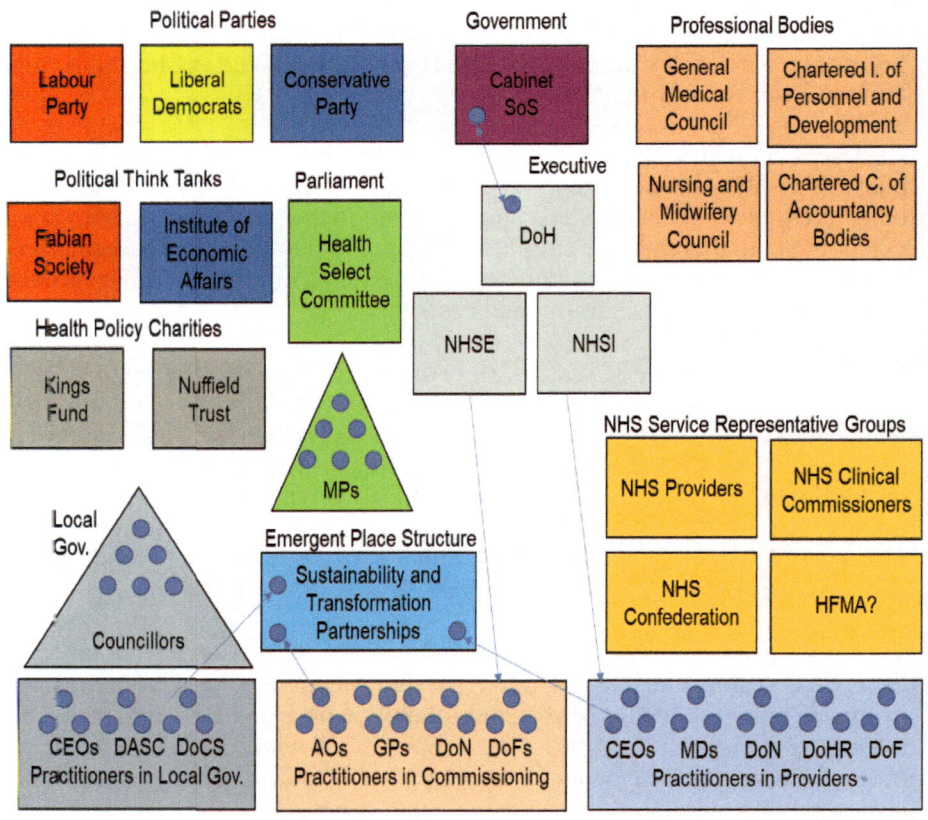

How it is possible to influence policy is therefore open to question. There are practitioners in local government, commissioning and provider organisations in the health and care system, who were participating in the emergent non-statutory structures associated with the Sustainability and Transformation Partnerships and are now making sense of the consequences of the 2022 Act. There were and are local government councillors, as well as officers engaged via the Health and Well-Being Boards. Elsewhere, there are a range of NHS Service Representative Groups, such as the NHS Confederation, NHS Providers and the NHS Clinical Commissioners. Here we might also position HFMA, as a representative body of NHS finance. There is not an equivalent representative body of NHS nurses, doctors or HR practitioners, in quite the same way. The professional bodies for these professions are also shown above. It may be worthy of note that there is not now a particularly active NHS general management association. There was previously a relatively active Institute of Health Service Management, but it is not as active as it once was, and this could explain the reasons why the practitioner voice in policy change and adoption may be weak and has not managed to generate a policy alternative to the internal market.

Beyond these bodies within and representing the system, there was the Department of Health, NHSI and NHSE which can be regarded as the executive function of the English NHS from a policy delivery perspective. The Department is led by the Secretary of State for Health, who creates the connection into Government, which is where health policy could be regarded as fundamentally determined - either explicitly through the manifesto commitments of the three major political parties in England, or non-manifesto commitments, either via statute law, or executive orders. MP oversight comes from the Health Select Committee which has been cited within the thesis. Then there is a series of politically aligned think tanks, such as the Fabian Society and the Institute of Economic Affairs, representing the political left and right, respectively. There are also some non-politically aligned health-specific think tanks within the health system, such as the Kings' Fund and Nuffield Trust.

The role of ideas in the policy process (John, 1998; Baggot, 2007) in explaining policy change and policy persistence is key from the author's perspective. Where the policy community is currently at in negotiating and grappling with public policy ideas, and whether a consensus view exists is important, for the policy process and policy adoption. For a top-down view of the policy position, it is possible to review the manifestos of the main parties in the last three general elections, which are shown in Table 6.1 below. There was a reference in all the general election manifestos by the three main English parties in 2015 and 2017 on health service organisation, competition and to some extent the internal market. But, by 2019 only the Liberal Democrats mentioned reforming

NHS structures. The lack of the Conservative and Labour reference in 2019 could be due to there being a broader political divergence between the Johnson-led and the Corbyn-led parties.

Table 6.1 – 2015, 2017 and 2019 Conservative, Labour and Liberal Democrat Manifesto References to NHS Structural Reform

Conservative – 2015 - We will continue to integrate the health and social care systems, joining-up services between homes, clinics and hospitals, including through piloting new approaches like the pooling of around £6 billion of health and social care funding in Greater Manchester and the £5.3 billion Better Care Fund. (The Conservative Party (2015); 39)
Conservative – 2017 - We will hold NHS England's leaders to account for delivering their plan to improve patient care. If the current legislative landscape is either slowing implementation or preventing clear national or local accountability, we will consult and make the necessary legislative changes. This includes the NHS's own internal market, which can fail to act in the interests of patients and creates costly bureaucracy. So, we will review the operation of the internal market and, in time for the start of the 2018 financial year, we will make non-legislative changes to remove barriers to the integration of care. (The Conservative Party (2015); 67)
Labour – 2015 - The answer to the health challenges we face is not to set hospital against hospital, but to join up services around patients' needs. We will repeal the Government's Health and Social Care Act, scrapping the competition regime and restoring proper democratic accountability for the NHS. We will establish a sensible commissioning framework, based on the principle of an NHS preferred provider, to stop the drive towards privatisation and make sure that NHS services are not destabilised by competition and fragmentation. Commissioning and budgets will be brought together at a local level to join up services and make sure that providers are incentivised to help people stay healthy and outside hospital, rather than simply waiting for them to fall ill. (The Labour Party (2015); 34 and 35)

Table 6.1 - continued

Labour – 2017 - Labour will halt and review the NHS 'Sustainability and Transformation Plans', which are looking at closing health services across England, and ask local people to participate in the redrawing of plans with a focus on patient need rather than available finances. We will create a new Quality, safety and excellence regulator – to be called 'NHS Excellence'.

The next Labour government will reverse privatisation of our NHS and return our health service into expert public control. Labour will repeal the Health and Social Care Act that puts profits before patients and make the NHS the preferred provider. We will reinstate the powers of the Secretary of State for Health to have overall responsibility for the NHS. (The Labour Party (2017); 69)

Liberal Democrat – 2015 - Secure local agreement on full pooling of budgets between the NHS and care services with a target date of 2018, consulting on a legal duty for this. The details of how services are commissioned will remain a matter for local areas. In this way we will build on the radical proposals to integrate health and care funding in Greater Manchester.

Continue to develop Health and Wellbeing Boards to take a broad view of how services can improve wellbeing in their area, ensuring democratic accountability for local care.

Liberal Democrats are committed to repealing any parts of the Health and Social Care Act 2012 which make NHS services vulnerable to forced privatisation through international agreements on free markets in goods and services. We will end the role of the Competition and Markets Authority in health, making it clear that the needs of patients, fairness and access always come ahead of competition, and that good local NHS services do not have to be put out to tender. (The Liberal Democrat Party (2015); 73)

Table 6.1 - continued

Liberal Democrat – 2017 - Establish a cross-party health and social care convention, bringing together stakeholders from all political parties, patients' groups, the public and professionals from within the health and social care system to carry out a comprehensive review of the longer-term sustainability of the health and social care finances and workforce, and the practicalities of greater integration. We would invite the devolved administrations to be a part of this work.

We need services that fit around people's lives, not ones that force them to fit their lives around the care they need. This will become increasingly important as our population ages and the number of people living with long-term conditions grows. It is also more cost-effective to support people to be able to live at home rather than endure lengthy stays in hospital. We must move away from a fragmented system to an integrated service with more joined-up care and more personal budgets so that people can design services for their own individual needs. We believe this should happen from the bottom up, suiting the needs of local communities.

Remodel the health care funding system to eliminate perverse incentives, by moving away from payments for activity and introducing tariffs that encourage joined-up services and promote improved outcomes for patients and better preventive care. (The Liberal Democrat Party (2017); 17 and 20)

Liberal Democrat – 2019 - Support the changes to the Health and Social Care Act recommended by the NHS, with the objective of making the NHS work in a more efficient and joined-up way, and to end the automatic tendering of services. (The Liberal Democrat Party (2019); 58)

In the manifestos in both 2015 and 2017, the author would claim there was a degree of at least rhetorical alignment around the three main political parties in the UK, surrounding the need for integration, and not letting the internal market get in the way of that. There was perhaps also a bit of political point scoring from Labour on the STPs, but not a substantial policy divergence. There was a stated aim from the Conservatives on removing the barriers to integration, and a stated aim from the Liberal Democrats on the need to ensure there is cross-party support not only on the financial settlement but also on the way to further integrate structures, including the devolved nations. The Conservative and Labour manifestos in 2019 spoke far more of spending and priorities, as opposed to how the NHS should be organised. The Liberal Democrats were explicit about their support for the NHSE/I proposals to bring about legislative change to integrate structures in 2019. Even though the Conservative manifesto did not mention this support, they have agreed with the recommendation by bringing forward the Health and Care Act 2022.

Marking the 70th Anniversary of the NHS in 2018, there have been some updates from some of the political think tanks and interest groups. The IEA (Niemietz, 2018) notes, slightly off-beam from the three main parties' manifestos, and wider commentary and mainstream opinion:

> 2002 onwards saw a re-emergence of the market mechanisms in the NHS, following attempts to create an internal market in the 1990s. A new payment mechanism was gradually introduced, patients were given a choice of provider at the point of referral, and providers were given greater autonomy. There were also efforts to strengthen the role of commissioners and make use of private capital in the building and maintenance of new healthcare facilities. Empirical evidence from the 'quasi-market' reform period is overwhelmingly positive, and these reforms should be built upon to improve patient choice, strengthen the self-governance of providers and enshrine the principle that the money follows the patient. (Niemietz (2018); 9).

This author would question whether the evidence from "quasi-market" reform was overwhelmingly positive. The Fabian Society (Kerslake, 2018), a Labour policy group, unsurprisingly, has a slightly different perspective:

> A huge simplification and reduction in costly bureaucracy could be achieved by moving away from the current commissioner provider split at a local level and introducing long-term 10-year contracts based on the size and needs of the local population. More of the NHS commissioning budget, for example for mental health services, could be determined locally. There should be the opportunity to reconfigure clinical commissioning group boundaries to better align with those of local government. (Kerslake, 2018: 37).

A more politically centralist perspective may be gained from a Civitas report, containing commentaries from both Paul Corrigan and Stephen Dorrell (see Stubbs, 2018):

> Getting patient care organised around the patient and not the existing NHS organisation will take a shift in power...For this, active patients will need new organisations that will take the lead in coordinating what are, at present, fragmented NHS institutions and working beyond the NHS with social care and other support from the voluntary sector. (Stubbs, 2018: 121).

> Indeed, it is often argued that 'there is no evidence that commissioning adds value and it is time to recognise that it has failed'. The problem with this argument is that its proponents have nothing to put in its place. (Stubbs, 2018: 130).

Despite the broad political consensus on the need for further integration and a questioning of the need for an internal market mechanism, there is a continuing policy divergence on the precise way in which that is done and then implemented. The author, therefore, in terms of his own sphere of influence, has initially concentrated his efforts on trying to change the system from within, either via his previous NHSI role or previous role within the Derbyshire STP, or via the utilisation of the HFMA, as the representative group of NHS finance practitioners, via its Policy and Research Committee. He has also become involved in change projects, such as that with PwC. There is not a policy consensus on the way to organise the system differently, which, to some extent, has delivered a continuation of the status quo since 2012. But there is the opportunity for the author to try and validate his own views on the system by challenging them, and then honing them further, amongst fellow practitioners, before trying to influence the complex policy network that exists, relating to the English NHS and its finances.

Whether this work within HFMA and elsewhere will directly influence policy is debatable, though, due to the potentially diffuse nature and complexity of the policy-making process, the multiple stakeholders associated with developing and delivering policy, and the potential absence of a consensus around the precise route to take to try and re-organise the English NHS. It could be this complexity and the lack of a consensus around ideas that ultimately reduce practitioner participation in the policy development process. However, despite the ex-ante belief that action research may not initially deliver a transformative jump in the policy consensus around the internal market, this should not necessarily be a cause for concern. This thesis could just be a case study which is trying to understand how practitioners influence policy. Exworthy et al (2012: 234) described:

> The value of case studies is both to shed light on empirical phenomenon and to offer insights into theoretical statements. However, as case

studies illustrate policy evolution and change over time, they can also provide opportunities for learning – the way in which we understand learning in theory and practice.

6.2 Overview and Role of Action Research

Given that the third Research Question relates to the ability of practitioners to influence policy this aims to be an action research element of the project. As just described immediately above the impact of that action could be somewhat diffused and less than hoped for but change is the intent. A description by Bowling (2009: 441) noted:

> Action research is undertaken by participants in social situations to improve their practices and their understanding of them. The method was designed to study social systems with the aim of changing them (i.e., to achieve certain goals). It is a community-based method.

The stages of action research defined by Stringer (2007), involve:

> 1) Setting the Stage – which the author believes he has done via the joint HFMA and PwC work and HFMA involvement in the Policy and Research Committee and Trustee.
>
> 2) Looking – the facilitator must next enable participants jointly to describe the situation and the problem, made possible by the approach to the HFMA/PwC report and also the work in the Policy and Research Committee.
>
> 3) Thinking - the facilitator plans to organise meetings that enable participants to understand and interpret the situation, described in the next section of this chapter, and beyond that within the HFMA.
>
> 4) Acting – the solutions to the problem should be planned by all the stakeholder groups, which is more complex in the context of this project due to the complexity of the multiple stakeholders described in Figure 6.1.

Table 6.2 - Action Research Questionnaire (Hart and Bond (1995))

Question 1 – What is the purpose of the proposed project?

The project is trying to influence policy around the NHS internal market in the English NHS. It is trying to engage practitioners in finance in health to develop thinking around how we change and modify the way the system is managed, structured and financed.

Question 2 – Why is it important to do something about this situation at this point in time?

There is currently a wider policy and political debate about the amount of money the English NHS needs. Also, there is a debate about how the NHS in England continues to be organised with a purchaser/provider split, which many believe is not in the best interest of patients. Emergent non-statutory structures called Sustainability and Transformation Partnerships are being formed to try and address systems planning more effectively together, but these structures are not a legal entity and are not fully addressing some of the divisions in the system.

Question 3 – Why do you want to initiate such a project?

I have worked in NHS finance for 25 years and am also a Trustee of an organisation called the Healthcare Finance Management Association. I think as a finance professional in health we should be contributing to how we should change the system, as many of us do not feel it is adequate or fit for purpose.

Question 4 – Is there a problem (that is, an expression of a need for change) and, if so, who says there is?

In a recent HFMA/PWC survey of 203 finance practitioners in health, 76% believed the current approach to funding NHS organisations was not fit for purpose, 83% believed there was a conflict between long term financial sustainability and short term savings, 80% believed there should be a single budget for each local health, social care and public health economy, and over 70% believed an integrated system will produce better value for money for patients.

The author has used the Hart and Bond (1995) Self-Assessment questionnaire to try and describe the purpose of the action research more precisely. The first four questions from this questionnaire, and the author's answers, are shown in Table 6.2. This starts to give a framework to the third research aim around influencing, seeking views, understanding and structuring finance practitioner views in health to influence the policy landscape.

In moving to describe the action research associated with the project, the author believed he had captured practitioner views, and validated conclusions from Chapter 5 on the difficult status of the NHS provider and wider English NHS financial system and the approach to the internal market. This enabled him to question and require fundamental changes to the current working of the NHS. However, these are contested findings, as noted by McNiff et al (2003: 129):

> When you say you have learned something, you are making a claim that you know something that was not known before. This is your original claim to knowledge. If the knowledge is to be taken seriously as knowledge, and not opinion or conjecture, it has to be validated; that is, agreed by someone else to be justifiably believable. Doing this can be problematic, because not all participants may agree on what counts as valid knowledge, and which criteria and standards of judgements should be used in coming to this decision.

The social intent of the research is to improve the situation the English NHS finds itself in, noting the lack of a precise consensus on the policy's next steps to address this. This is being performed by making some of the tacit knowledge of the author explicit, both via the professional doctoral process and via his activity within the Policy and Research Committee and Trustee role in the HFMA and his role on CIPFA Council and within the Public Policy and Reform Faculty Board. The more difficult element of the action research aim of the project is to demonstrate clearly how the action research phase has met the social intent, particularly in a policy context.

Figure 6.2 - Summary Sphere of Influence: Changing the Internal Market - Allies, Opponents and Neutrals (Hart and Bond, 1995)

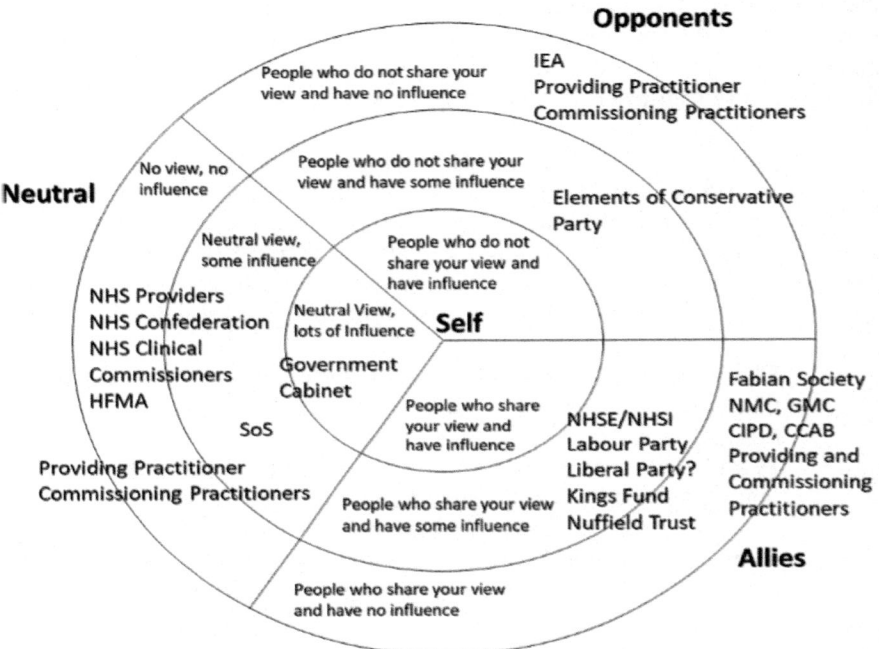

Beyond getting a good insight into practitioner views in NHS finance, the author has started to address why the policy environment may be hard to influence, as shown in Figure 6.3, as part of the Hart and Bond questionnaire. This shows which stakeholders may be allies or opponents of change. There are more allies, but the author has noted that practitioners working in the system may be allies, opponents or neutrals. It is perhaps this practitioner fragmentation that has contributed to the internal market remaining longer than opinions and policy evidence suggested sensible.

6.3 Overview of Findings on Healthcare Funding and Practitioner Views via the HFMA Policy and Research Committee

The results of the regression analysis work and the key findings from the HFMA/PwC, "Making Money Work in the Health and Care System", were discussed within the Policy and Research Committee of the HFMA. The Terms of Reference of the Policy and Research Committee are orientated unsurprisingly towards influencing the UKs health policy and researching in the NHS finance arena to deliver this aim. This was the main group used to pursue the action research phase of the project. A key challenge for the author was to define the exit point from this group, in terms of completing the professional doctorate, whilst this work inevitably continues beyond the precise confines of this thesis.

The Policy and Research Committee, like the HFMA, itself, is composed of stakeholders, representing all views from within the NHS finance function, so like the Stakeholder Group for the HFMA/PwC work, they would be a good group to potentially pursue the "Looking, Thinking and Acting" phases of the action research. There are representatives of providers, commissioners, NHSI, NHSE, Department of Health and the National Audit Office. The Terms of Reference of the group explicitly include providing a forum for discussing healthcare finance policy and agreeing on HFMA's policy views, overseeing the development of the HFMA's policy and technical work programme, commissioning and/or co-ordinating research, co-ordination of policy and research activities of local HFMA groups, and providing advice and guidance on how the HFMA should respond to consultation responses and submissions to Parliamentary Committees.

The agenda and minutes of the meetings of the Policy and Research Committee on 13th February and 22nd May 2018 are shown in Appendices 8 to 11. A presentation was used to inform the group on the research findings in Chapters 3 and 4. A transcript of the 40 minutes discussion, held at the meeting, was then used to review and evaluate the discussions.

The nature of the discussions of the Policy and Research Committee was helpful and productive. There was a review of the presentation produced from both the regression work and the HFMA/PwC report, and the conclusions made in response related both to a) challenging and contributing to methodology, and b) suggestions for further work/analysis. In general, there was a more heated conversation related to the regression work and a more reconciled response to the HFMA/PwC report "Making Money Work in the Health and Care System".

The initial challenge to the regression analysis related to the financial performance of Trusts and the extent to which the reported financial positions were truly reflective of the underlying performance. The reported positions include a number of non-recurrent items, such as the inclusion of profits on asset disposal, and other technical items, and it was not possible to easily separate out all the non-recurrent items, which was a noted methodological concern, which may be understating the actual overall size and problem of the deficits within provider finances, which have been described earlier in the thesis.

The second concern related to the approach to measuring the reference cost index. This can either be measured by adjusting for the Market Forces Factor or not. It was explained that the analysis used the unadjusted positions as we were separately looking at the MFF as a potential causal factor of financial performance as an independent variable. The reason why this is contentious links to the extent to which the MFF is truly a good and appropriate measure of regional variations in costs. One of the members of the group represented a provider with a very low MFF, so was particularly interested in this point.

The next methodological conversation related to the complexity of mapping the provider positions to the commissioner positions. Within the utilised methodology the main commissioner relationship was mapped to each provider. The wider mapping of the precise connection between providers and commissioners is far more complicated than this simple mapping would suggest. Some providers just operate with one main commissioner, while others have a one-to-many relationship and therefore it would be possible to do further work on this mapping if the results were to be made more robust. This conversation continued into the area of noticing two quite different groupings of Trusts, i.e., one with a large commissioning base and one with a more direct set of relationships with commissioners, and the group wondered if it would be worth reviewing their financial performance separately.

A further substantive funding conversation related to the centrality of the reference cost index link to financial performance. If there is an internal market which is seeking to reward providers who manage to improve costs appropriately to do better than tariffs, this link is important. There was also a conversation around whether the cost per Weighted Activity Unit (WAU) – a new equivalent to the RCI, was correlated to RCI and whether that would be a useful piece of further work to check this. In this area though, it was asserted that if it wasn't possible to see a good RCI to good financial performance link it could be contended that it:

> ...actually, it gets to the heart of whether this is an expenditure problem within a provider or whether it is the tariff that's irredeemably broken. (Verbatim comment from 22nd May Policy and Research Committee)

This direct quote from the group questions the extent to which the current episodic payment mechanism is fit for purpose. If the Trusts with better unit costs were not being incentivised by, and performing better under the current tariff mechanism, then the internal market may be seen to have a significant problem. The next conversation discussed whether there is a correlation between RCI and financial performance, and financial performance versus the nature and the blend and type of clinical work being performed at a hospital.

If an organisation undertakes much-unscheduled care activity, seen to be less financially advantageous, this can force organisations to leave elective capacity unutilised, driving poor financial performance potentially outside the organisation's control.

The debate on the trusts that had diversified their income streams and therefore looked to be more successful was of interest to the Policy and Research Committee. It was sensibly contended that this was leaving Trusts without these activities at a disadvantage. Essentially the surpluses against these alternative activities may be acting as an overall deflator to actual NHS healthcare tariffs. So those that were predominantly delivering NHS treatment and care (the majority of Trusts) were potentially suffering at the hands of a minority of Trusts, who had been able to earn a good income from someone or somewhere else. This was also believed to challenge the overall tariff-setting methodology, because this was seen to deflate the overall reference cost quantum, in the same way as income from education and research may be deflating it. More generally, this led to a debate about tariff setting and the fact that the overall income to Trusts was felt to be always capped from the centre to the current income quantum, not necessarily the costs of service delivery.

Beyond the modelling work performed on the different levels of capital in each Trust derived from a PFI source, the Committee believed that further work could be of interest to look at the precise structure of each PFI scheme. The nature of each PFI scheme could be reviewed concerning whether there were both soft and/or hard Facilities Management with them and the nature of the RPI inflator within the contracts was thought to be the larger determinant of financial performance within PFI schemes, not just the underlying capital cost, which was measured within the regression analysis.

The results for the CQC and Emergency Department (ED) performance and the correlation with financial performance were discussed. It was thought credible that additional quality performance was not necessarily costing additional money. The Committee discussed ED performance is a good barometer of flow through the hospital, meaning by doing better at managing unscheduled care as a system, you'd then be more likely to be delivering more financially advantageous elective work and not taking "a hit" on elective delivery. Those better able to manage unscheduled care would have better provider income.

A suggestion which was made at the meeting of the Policy and Research Committee on 13th February 2018 related to the potential correlation between stable leadership in organisations and systems, and its correlation to the broader and financial health of organisations. Again, this claim was made on 22nd May, which was further elaborated upon in terms of those areas that had stable leadership, as that generated the right system-level working through trust within those systems. Again, it was considered difficult to measure but there was a good deal of positive support for this claim.

There was also an assertion that financial performance was reviewed with reference to the speed with which each Trust had achieved Foundation Trust (FT) status by looking at when they received FT status (as part of which wave). Originally, FT status had been awarded based on an assessment process strongly geared towards financial health. These were thought to always have been the higher financially performing organisations with better than average strength of cash and balance sheet positions which would have been those that achieved FT status earlier. It was also thought sensible to look at particular Trusts by type, (i.e., acute, community, mental health); and where possible to examine the more precise case-mix and service type analysis within each Trust, to see if that was a cause of financial health.

Turning to the discussion relating to the HFMA/PwC report on practitioner views, and whether there was anything contentious within it, no one believed there was. Perhaps mirroring the party-political consensus from the 2015 and 2017 manifestos, all the shorter-term and longer-term recommendations in the report were broadly supported. It was noted that it was perhaps unsurprising that personal health budgets had not received much backing from the provider reference group polling. This item and proposition, personal health budgets, were perhaps more of a commissioning than a provisioning issue.

The conversation then moved on and noted that systems were already underway developing a different financial framework than the national one. One example was jointly being developed between two providers and one commissioner, to get to a cost-based focus on system savings, in a particular STP area. Others noted that the precise nature of the national financial framework and specifically contractual forms haven't inhibited local systems from defining local approaches moving away from the national policy mainstream in NHS system management and finance. Fundamentally, it was generally believed that there was a national framework and management model for the English NHS, but there were many local variations and hidden complexities in the English NHS finance system, making a nationwide analysis even more complicated.

All the participants in the Committee on 22nd May volunteered to contribute to the then-proposed semi-structured interviews on practitioner influence on policy, as did some of the members of the committee, who had not been able to attend.

6.4 Summary on the Impact of Evidence and Practitioner Views on NHS Finance and Internal Market Policy

Given that the whole of the Policy and Research Committee was happy to further participate in the research associated with this thesis, the author decided to test practitioner views on the practitioner role in policy and policy development, at the next meeting on 18th September 2018, as opposed to the previously posited route of a series of individual semi-structured interviews. This had several advantages from the author's perspective: it would take less time, would ensure continued ownership of the work associated with the thesis within the HFMA, and was more reflective of the four steps identified by Stringer (2007), as a key part of the action research process and congruent with the overall "role-based emergent opportunism" approach.

As a consequence of this changed approach, the author notified HFMA of the need to put the research on the agenda. He then prepared a further presentation for the group. The minutes and the transcript of the meeting were then reviewed and descrbed. The group which met on 18th September 2018 had seven of the ten participants that had been at the May meeting. There were then a further three participants who had not been at the May meeting. For the benefit of those three, there was a reasonable time spent at the start of the September Policy and Research agenda item, recapping the previous conversation.

Following Baggot (2007) and his five views on policy implementation, there was a discussion on the different views of policy implementation in the context of health policy. Responses from the group concentrated on their role in policy design and how to best implement policy. The discussion in the group dealt with the large issues in policy, such as the nature of whether we had a purchaser/provider split in health, and that this had arrived as part of a political narrative from a hierarchical source. It was noted that the ability for us as practitioners to call for the end of the internal market was considerably easier now, as there was such consensus for the need for this policy change.

There was then a discussion on the nature of the over-riding policy imperative regarding the "NHS free at the point of need" and that at some points perhaps this huge policy imperative did not allow for the appropriate conversation about how much that might cost, in a changing environment, both in terms of population and technology. There was also a conversation about the nature of the regional politics in Northern Ireland, Scotland and Wales, enabling an earlier rejection of the internal market due to the political consensus being slightly more to the left than England. There was then a discussion on the extent to which we were already adapting the English market policy due to the introduction of the STPs. A further discussion about the institutional and individual biases in the system to potentially maintain the status quo also ensued.

The backing for the need to replace the internal market was reinforced following the discussion of the Ideas contained in the three main Party Manifestos in 2015 and 2017. The reflections on manifestos, from a practitioner perspective, were broadly along the lines of how the Conservatives had perhaps moved a little leftwards in their narrative about the NHS, and how STP-related developments were ensuring that the NHS debate was becoming overtly more connected to the political process. This connection to the political process was noted in Wales and Greater Manchester, where local politicians were thought to be more overtly engaged and supportive in those differing structures. The policy was not thought too political for practitioners to engage in, but there was an appreciation of the need to ensure that the practitioners in the NHS, like the civil service more generally, were helping to appropriately implement policy, and remain able to work with all political parties when they were in government.

There were some mixed responses to the proposals of Paton (2016) for a tidied-up NHS (Table 2.2) on the precise way of changing the internal market structures. There was a view expressed about the centrality of hospitals to the system and in the public consciousness. The extent to which building a new system around the hospital infrastructures may not precipitate the changes in out-of-hospital care that some of the group thoughts were necessary. There was also the view expressed that having a more separate set of mental health providers may reinforce the need to ensure that mental health was seen with equal parity.

The role of GPs was discussed and where they should fit in the system. In response to the question as to whether we needed to revert to a system that looked more like the District Health Authority structure of pre-1989 or not, there was a view that we should not go back to an identical system, although there were benefits. The discussion then turned to the extent to which the structure became a function of the level of growth of funding that the system received. If higher growth, an internal market looked more tenable, if very flat funding, possibly not. Indeed, there was a view that the relative success of the structures may have had more to do with funding growth into the system at the time, as opposed to the relative merits or disadvantages of the structures themselves.

Following the completion of the Hart and Bond questionnaire, the author prepared a force field analysis on the internal market, based on the work by Lewin, as described in Stacey (1993), to try and explain the factors which were driving and inhibiting changes to the system:

> Lewin (1947) saw social planning as a means of improving the functioning of organisations. He saw social planning processes in terms of circular feedback in which goals were clarified, paths identified, and actions kept to the path, through the option of negative feedback. (Stacey, 1993; 135).

Figure 6.3 - Force Field Analysis Developed by the Author on the Internal Market

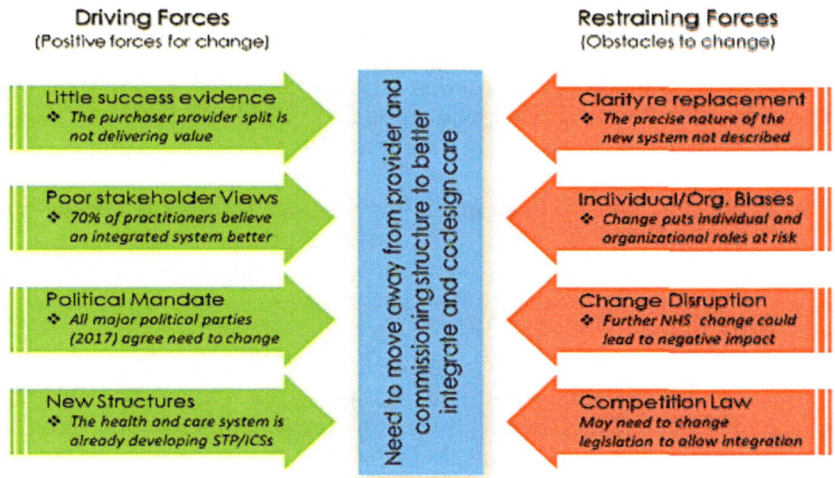

Lewin thought of organisational change around a) initially systems being in a state of equilibrium, with b) driving change and resisting forces balancing each other, which are then c) potentially triggered by something than imbalances, which d) causes a search for a new recipe to seek balance during a reformulation period, which then e) eventually leads to a system refreezing as the forces rebalance around that new recipe. Through his research and reflective practice, the author has identified four driving forces for change around changing from the NHS internal market; i) little success evidence, ii) poor stakeholder views, iii) a political mandate and iv) emergent new structures; and, four restraining factors keeping the internal market in place, i) the clarity on the replacement or a new recipe, ii) individual and organisational change biases, iii) the fear of further change disruption and iv) the need to change the application of competition law to the NHS.

In response to the force field analysis, the group largely agreed on the factors that were leaving the NHS internal market in a balanced force field. They also recognised the need for a new recipe but didn't see us yet entering the 'reformulation' or 'refreezing' stages. The initial response to the force field analysis, related to the third restraining force associated with the change disruption and how the change from PCTs to CCGs had seen a loss of relationships between providers and commissioners which in the view of the Committee had impacted negatively on the system. In conclusion, the force field analysis received broad support. The discussion then moved onto the nature of the current government, the inability to find a 'new recipe' and the lack of legislative time or support to bake that recipe. The committee broadly agreed that the consequence of this was that we were 'stuck with a system that doesn't work and a load of workarounds' (Verbatim comment from 18th September Policy and Research Committee).

This conclusion adheres to a view that has been established in public policy that the current policy is very dependent on the preceding policy and is said to be path dependent as described by Kay et al (2013: 464).

> Path dependency is an appealing concept for understanding public policy development; it provides a label for the observations and intuitions that policies, once established, can be difficult to change or reform.

Perhaps a telling but unspoken reason for the practitioners in the NHS finance community continuing to support the nature of the extant internal market structure of the English NHS is the fact that they inhabited it. Although the author thinks the new public management view of the public bureaucracy (Niskanen, 1971) overstates the self-interest of those in the public sector, it would be difficult to imagine that practitioners would advocate strongly to "topple the structure" that they inhabited, without noting the potential consequence on them, if the structure they inhabited and operated, were collapsed or replaced.

For the author to change and provoke thinking about NHS reforms, he has written blogs on the Healthcare Financial Management Association's website, such as Outhwaite (2012), and now sits on both the governing bodies of HFMA and CIPFA to try and influence national policymaking. The author, therefore, seeks to describe and develop a debate on the impact of markets and competition on the English NHS. He has also lectured internationally on health service finance and is engaged in work with the US, Australia and The Netherlands to compare and contrast different approaches to financial management in health.

The starting point of the approach to the dissemination strategy for the research findings will be via the HFMA. Throughout the thesis, the author sought to make recommendations on improvements to the systems in place. The research aimed to influence the approach in his field directly and to contribute to the specific debate on NHS markets and provide an example of practitioner research in NHS finance at doctoral level, and to support work he is also engaged in on the HFMAs Finance MBA. For this reason, the research adopted an action research approach. The Hart and Bond (1995) self-assessment questionnaire, particularly seek to clarify the researcher's thinking about the purpose, timing, initiation and need for the research.

> It is designed to assist with thinking about the research project and the context of the proposed piece of research. It draws on practice wisdom, your own knowledge of the setting in which you work and your own methods, actual and potential. It also prompts you to consider ways in which you might be able to generate qualitative and quantitative data from everyday activities to help in analysing the problem and the context, and includes practical suggestions for ways in which you might undertake some fact-finding. (Hart and Bond, 1995: 186)

If we now revisit the role of the epistemic community in English NHS finance it is worth noting and describing its different roles. Certainly, there is a pure implementation role, but there are those within that community who wish to influence policy direction and try to improve the policy itself. Some policies do arrive top-down, but the policy can be influenced and directed in a particular way, which was seen as the internal market NHS policy from very early in its development.

The internal market policy for "Market 1" and "Market 2" can be seen using the McConnell (2010) framework, described in section 2.8, perhaps as delivering i) little societal benefit, or ii) public value. It probably iii) didn't show an evidenced approach to good practice, despite observing a trend for markets in public policy, but iv) did probably accrue benefits to political actors on both sides evidencing an approach to trying to deliver productivity and effectiveness. In truth, and certainly by "Market 3", the policy was v) delivering only marginal success, (but this wasn't well acknowledged), if any success at all, and was beginning to show vi) failure and fiasco.

By the time of the 2022 Act, the a) policy process was slowly getting even more derailed and side-lined (particularly during the pandemic), and b) the rationale for the programme was increasingly contested or not understood, and therefore by 2019, c) the politics were becoming unsuccessful, and a replacement largely supported.

Based on McConnell's (2010) analysis, definitions of political success, the internal market policy could increasingly be seen to be at best, a conflicted success in various dimensions, by the time of the 2022 Act, as shown in Table 6.3, populated by the author. The author doesn't see the policy process, programme or politics of the internal market over the different measures of success as any better than a conflicted success, by the time of the 2022 Act. The processes within it were at best a precarious success. The programme itself was a conflicted success. From the 2012 Act onwards the politics of the policy approach had brought the NHS internal market into fiasco territory, in terms of the views at the time, and then beyond the legislative "pause". The manifestos in 2015, 2017 and 2019 certainly not identify the internal market approach as a potential political success.

Table 6.3 – Internal Market Policy Success by the time of the 2022 Act, populated by the author, using McConnell's (2010) approach.

	Process	**Programme**	**Politics**
Social Benefit	Precarious success	Conflicted Success	Failure
Public Value	Precarious success	Conflicted Success	Failure
Good Practice policymaking	Precarious success	Conflicted Success	Failure
Accruing benefit to Political Actors	Failure	Failure	Failure
Policy success only marginal	Failure	Failure	Failure
Avoids Fiasco/Failure	Failure	Failure	Failure

This chapter has reviewed the changing views of the internal market over time. At the time of a pre-progression pilot study, there was some, but not whole-hearted, support for the internal market. The fact that there was some support within the system for the internal market for a time is of interest. If the policy was set up as a response to challenge the monopolistic provision of NHS services (Tullock, 2000; Niskanen, 1971), and challenge the very bureaucrats that inhabited that system, it could be questioned why there should have been any support at all, if those policy aims were understood within the system.

After the 2012 Act and subsequent events, there was less support from NHS finance practitioners and wider groups for the internal market, evidenced by the HFMA/PwC report and the subsequent HFMA Policy and Research Committee discussions, and then wider sources. There was not however a consensus on what to replace the NHS internal market with and therefore we are in a policy held within the described balanced force field, that has been generated by the path dependency of NHS policy since 1989. How the Health and Care Act 2022 is interpreted and implemented will be the next critical phase of the English NHS's organisational development, and whether we fully shake off the internal market through this process awaits to be seen.

CHAPTER 7

CONCLUSIONS, RECOMMENDATIONS AND PROPOSED FURTHER RESEARCH

This chapter provides a summary of the issues raised and addressed, in answer to the three Research Questions, stated in Section 1.1, which have been addressed in chapters 4, 5 and 6. This chapter then draws together the overall themes from the research and forms a conclusion on the overall internal market policy in the English NHS. It also presents a series of recommendations at a micro level (related to NHS finance), meso-level (related to the English NHS) and macro level (related to broader public policy). It then suggests some areas for further research, of which there are many - not least because of the potential inadequacy of the work undertaken, but also potentially because of the work's ambitious breadth.

7.1 Do Finance Practitioners believe the way the NHS is funded could run an internal market?

RQ1 evolved over time as described in Chapter 3. It moved from a view that an empirical study on the data could show whether the adequacy of the English NHS funding approach could run an internal market to an approach around whether practitioners in the English NHS finance thought that they were a street-level bureaucracy (Lipsky, 2010), and/or part of an Advocacy Coalition Framework (Weible, 2013) and/or an epistemic group (Haas, 2019); (concepts described in section 2.8); which would and could ensure the success of the NHS internal market. The views of Niskanen (1971) and Tullock (2000) (described in section 2.2) feel increasingly alien to the author, as the public sector seeks to find a departure from New Public Management and the internal market approach. Chapter 4 describes the approach to testing the primary research of the author around NHS funding with the HFMA Policy and Research Committee to see what this group thought about whether NHS funding could run a market and whether they believed that to be possible or desirable. Through the course of the research, as shown in Figure 3.3, much has changed over time, to try and resolve the internal market policy.

The results of the bivariate regression analysis of the financial performance of the 238 healthcare provider organisations financial performance and independent variables that could be causing such financial performance had two significant findings, in the opinion of the HFMA Policy and Research Committee. First, the absence of any correlation between lower unit costs in organisations and improved financial performance does call into question the nature of the approach we are pursuing in the pricing regime, to deliver an internal market mechanism. Second, the fact that the most significant correlation, for an independent variable, suggested that the higher the organisation had alternative income streams, the better they performed. These call into question the approach to core NHS funding for treatment and care. On this basis, it would be relatively hard to defend the statement that the funding approach was adequate to potentially change provision through a market mechanism. Of course, these results are contestable, and the further work performed on the multi-variate regression notes the difficulty in drawing absolute conclusions, as this second strand of statistical work shows. The view is that the funding was not appropriate to run a market broadly accepted by practitioners, both within the HFMA Policy and Research Committee and via the results of the HFMA/PwC survey work, however.

The work on this regression analysis perhaps does tell us it is possible to take a positivist stance on the adequacy of public policy, but this is a very complex area. It may be possible to challenge or support public policy from a positivist perspective, but it is very difficult. To make claims on the adequacy of policy without clearly identifying the ambiguities and irregularities in the policy landscape is difficult. The claims made via the regression analysis in this research are quite narrow and this analysis was used mainly to generate the Policy and Research Committee conversations. If the system is designed to try to incentivise financial delivery, to be cost competitive versus a nationally determined set of prices, and there is no correlation between unit costs and the financial performance of organisations, then the system would seem to be flawed. Equivalently, if one of the few ways for providers to make ends meet is to diversify, as the pricing mechanism seems unable to sustain the delivery of NHS services, that seems like an odd result, unless there was and is a stated aim for NHS provider organisations to diversify to subsidise NHS treatment and care. This might well be a sensible proposal, but it would need to be overtly stated in policy terms.

7.2 What are finance practitioners' views on the NHS internal market and what have the impact of those views been?

The approach to RQ2 also changed considerably over-time. The author's participation in the HFMA/PwC steering group was part of the "role-based emergent opportunism" approach described in section 3.8. This approach allowed a far bigger potential impact of the research, in terms of action research aims, and it also enabled a far broader approach to gathering data than would have been possible as an independent research-practitioner. There was a growing understanding of the need to understand theories of public policy implementation such as Pressman and Wildavsky (1973), Hill and Hupe

(2002), Matland (1995) and May and Winter (2007) described in Sections 2.7 and 2.8, to understand how the views of practitioners were impacting on policy success.

The additional approaches described in Chapter 5 to gauging practitioner views on the NHS internal market the data in the responses to the HFMA/PwC report being investigated via the NVivo coding of the responses was instructive to enable a deeper understanding of why the headline overall statistical findings in the report, that 70% of practitioners thought it was time for a policy change, was important. And as the party-political manifestos had all begun to suggest by 2017, most practitioners also backed a move towards an integrated system.

Based on the action research, undertaken beyond the HFMA/PwC report, via the HFMAs Policy and Research Committee, it was found that practitioners do understand the different policy drivers in the system but perhaps do not have the conceptual framework for anchoring the competing strands of English NHS policy, that the author's part-time, practitioner research has afforded him. As the participants in the HFMAs Policy and Research Committee are quite self-selecting in terms of their interests in policy and research a rich conversation ensued on the internal market policy. The HFMA Policy and Research Committee, therefore, perhaps had a heightened understanding than the wider practitioner body in NHS healthcare finance. The overall practitioner body research is likely to be more bounded than in the committee convenience sample. There are policy strands relating to, (i) market structures, (ii) targets, (iii) fundamental system thinking, (iv) management improvements and (v) wider public policy initiatives, is important, noted in section 3.1. These are all in play, and perhaps it requires a wider reading and understanding of NHS public policy and the origins of the internal market, to have a framework to interpret the overall policy environment fully. As not all members of the finance community of practice will have this wider perspective, therefore coming up with a definitive set of statements on the views of the community is hard. Notwithstanding these challenges, the HFMA/PwC report and the views of the policy research committee showed that an internal market was out of favour with finance practitioners. Although the HFMA/PwC report and the views of the Policy and Research Committee showed that an internal market was out of favour with finance practitioners, there was no consensus on the new recipe or replacement.

The motivations and beliefs of the practitioners in a system should not be underestimated in the context of the implementing policy. The approach to the development of the internal market has required a good deal of practitioner engagement and subsequent adaptation. Some have argued that adaptation began at the very outset of the policy. Now there is overwhelming support for change from several quarters without the right 'recipe' for the replacement being clear. Through the action research, there seems to be a high degree of understanding as much of the qualitative feedback in response to the HFMA/PwC open questions was very well considered. There is diminishing approval of the status quo as denoted by the very high percentages in the HFMA/PwC survey suggesting changes are required. There are also now overt adaptations in place, which means that the adoption of the policy on an internal market in health, is being actively circumvented, within the system itself locally, and via national interventions such as the development of the STPs, and the replacement of CCGs with ICBs, following the impact of the 2022 Act.

From the review of the responses by the HFMA Policy and Research committee, and in the experience of the author related to his wider HFMA, CIPFA and his current ICB role, there are interesting outstanding questions related to policy implementation success and the role of practitioners, their role as an epistemic community and the role of policy persistence and dependency, which are covered further in the Conclusions and Recommendations section. It is perhaps unsurprising that there is an inability to clearly define what the role of practitioners has been in the NHS internal market. On occasion the NHS finance community inhabits a position akin to the civil service, noting it is there to implement policy and not comment on it. Increasingly though there may be a growing need to comment on the adequacy of policy prior to implementation and this a growing call both within HFMA and CIPFA to advocate for policy that is more likely to deliver taxpayer and population value and that is more likely to succeed.

7.3 *How do Finance Practitioners Influence Policy?*

The role of the epistemic community (Haas, 2019) of NHS finance practitioners has not been actively and overtly researched by academic researchers in health policy. The author is firmly situated at a senior level as part of this epistemic group. The author finds himself increasingly advocating for a growing role in influencing policy for this epistemic group, due to his growing seniority, and growing belief that unless this group and the other coalitions of practitioners in the NHS believe in the public policy process and the policies being implemented, they are unlikely to work or succeed in delivering their stated aims. The idea of a neutral civil service role around policy implementation, for senior NHS finance practitioners (and wider NHS managerial and professional staff groups) who have seen NHS policy adoption through the front-line, irrespective of practitioner views of the potential efficacy of policy feels increasingly remote. Testing the thinking of the Policy and Research Committee of HFMA is an important attempt to try and understand how practitioners in NHS finance think they could and whether they should try to influence policy and this is discussed in Chapter 6.

Regardless of the opening evidence for the potential efficacy of the internal market in health, at the point of the inception of "Market 1" heralded by "Working for Patients", there seems to be little evidence of its success today, through the research approach adopted and in the opinion of the author. Opinion, as reflected in the HFMA/PwC (2018) report and the survey responses associated with it, and the discussions at the HFMA Policy and Research Committee, is now strongly weighted against the internal market's operation and, although there is no description of a clear alternative, work is underway to rectify this. This work will need to describe some clear policy next steps. The development of the response to the Health and Care Act (2022) will need to address the practical and policy issues associated with some of the frailties of the NHS internal market and deliver specific changes. At the moment practitioners are interpreting quite permissive primary legislation in the 2022 Act and are deviating from the old structures at different rates contingent on their views and the views of the ICBs and the various stakeholders in each of the ICPs. There is no common interpretation of the new English NHS system and a variety of views on what system changes would add the most value and give rise to the most public benefit. The debate on the best structure is to some extent being dwarfed by the more immediate challenges of workforce shortages and industrial action, the problems with the social care system and the large operational pressures the NHS and wider health and care system is experiencing in both unscheduled and scheduled care, post-pandemic.

The period from 2010 to the present day, has seen a further perpetuation of the internal market, even when evidence suggests this was not the appropriate policy. The "Never Again" 2012 Act (Timmins, 2012) can be seen as a particularly low point in the evidence-based approach. It is hard therefore to advocate for the point that policy is built from evidence. The author's force field analysis explains the perpetuation of the policy for longer than the policy evidence might have suggested and is due to the path dependency of the policy which is being changed by the Health and Care Act 2022. The muscle memory of the old system is hard to break, however, in the experience of the author in his new ICB role, the policy persistence concept feels highly prevalent.

The work of Baggot noting (i) policy as a rational, hierarchical process, (ii) policy borne of ideology and the interplay between ideas/concepts, political policies and public policy, versus (iii) policy as an interplay of interests and pressure groups, or (iv) policy determined via institutions and agendas or (v) policy as an adaptive learning process, does lend itself to a summary of these approaches in the context of the NHS internal market and health policy. There is, on occasion, in health policy i) a rational, hierarchical top-down view, but ii) sometimes the ideas and concepts underpinning policy are not clearly stated, neither are iii) the consequences of the interplay of interest and pressure groups on policy success stated, or are iv) how institutions and agendas are influencing that policy clearly stated, which often means that v) health policy always seems to feel like an adaptive learning process, from a practitioner perspective.

Figure 7.1 by the author links the politics of the internal market with the policy, its adoption, the required financial professional practice and then critical reflection. It also describes the antithesis to this system and the resultant critical reflections derived from some of the discussion at the September 2018 HFMA Policy and Research Committee, informed by the work of Mintzberg (2017), Fox (2018) and Seddon (2008). Figure 7.1 really polarises Cresswell (2009) "a basic set of beliefs that guide action" into two paradigms; "The internal market orthodoxy" - a more neo-liberal view of human action and the resultant policy; and "The antithesis – Planning" – more akin to the post-war settlement and health policy from 1948 to 1989, and perhaps where we are trying to return to, after the 2022 Act. Through his research the author has concluded the (i) post-positivism (determination, reductionism, empirical observation and measurement, and theory verification) is really hard to determine in terms of the effectiveness of health policy given the complexity of the system and the multiple levers being used to try and improve the approach, (ii) Social Constructivism (understanding, multiple participant meanings, social and historical construction and theory generation) seems a far more akin to how his view of the policy landscape is being determined and understood, (iii) Advocacy/participatory (political, empowered issue-orientated, collaborative and change-orientated) seems to describe a practical approach as to how to recommend next steps in the public policy landscape, and (iv) Pragmatism (consequences of actions, problem centred, pluralistic and real-world practice orientated) – seems valid, but there is a need to possibly describe from first principles how the policy actors are viewed within the systems to determine policy success.

Figure 7.1 - Politics, Policy, Adoption and Professional Practice in the NHS Internal Market

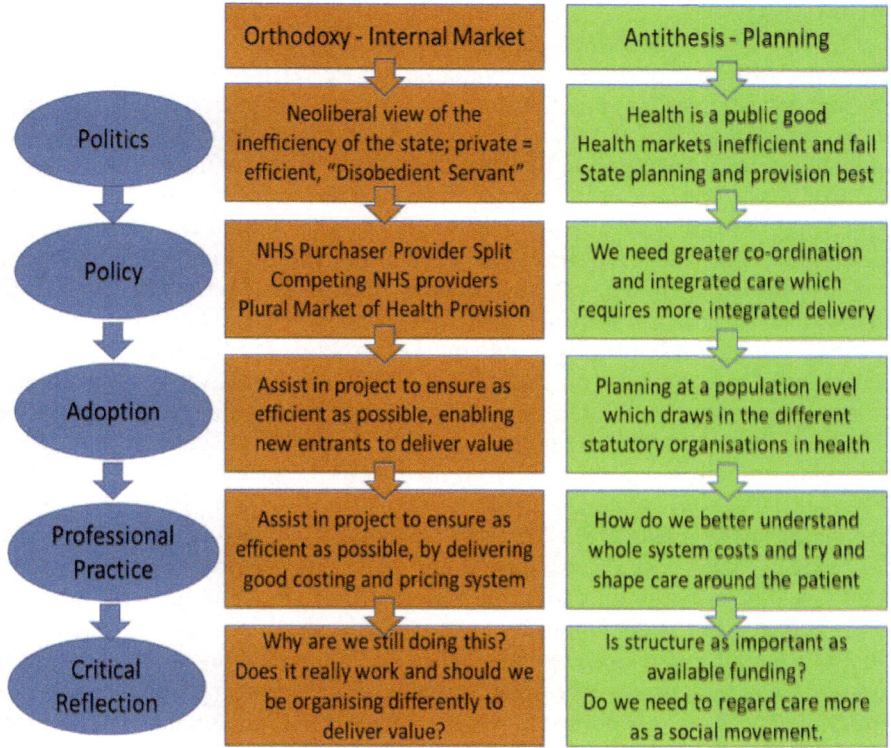

If policy actors are seen, to use the Le Grand (2003) terms, as "knightly" (Seddon (2008) a certain type of policy approach results which is more akin to that described in the "planning" paradigm. If policy actors are seen in a more "knave"- like way (Hayek (1944), Niskanen (1971) and Tullock (2000)) something more akin to the internal market approach results. On re-reading Cresswell's four definitions, having answered the research questions, the author has tried to make some firm conclusions and recommendations about the nature of the NHS quasi-market but does acknowledge the difficulty of observing the social phenomenon in this way, from a post-positivist perspective. His conclusions and recommendations position him more aligned to (Seddon 2008) as his practitioner view is that the internal market policy has given rise to many unintended consequences and has hampered actors within the system seeing the health and care system in a more integrated and unified way to deliver healthcare value in a more plural sense due to the policy fractures, identified in Chapter 1, between both provision and commissioning in the NHS, and between DHSC and DLUHC (and consequently local health bodies and local government).

There are different perspectives available on the NHS and the English NHS internal market, from (a) practitioner understanding and accounts, (b) real-time commentaries such as the Health Service Journal, (c) academic perspectives and (d) practitioner research. Practitioner research may be the bridge between some of these perspectives. The author would claim that the evidence for the effectiveness of the internal market in health has always been contested and that the original policy had a political antecedent in the New Public Management. It is difficult to find a cogent New Public Management rationalisation of the NHS internal market prior to 1989. Although not a new right author, Enthoven (1985) did tentatively propose some market structures in the NHS, but not the market we developed and now still have despite the 2022 Act. Enthoven was proposing competing healthcare management organisations, with integration between primary and secondary care, not the purchaser/provider split we have in England which separates GPs from the rest of the provision.

After over thirty years (1989-2022) of attempted changes to and move towards the internal market policy, advocated earlier in this period by a public policy coalition, it is probably time to try something different. Although a full revision to the antithesis of state planning seems unlikely, this planning approach is far closer to the language and the experience of this practitioner in recent years. His work as a practitioner, both nationally and in Derbyshire, and now South Yorkshire, is far more congruent with an approach of state planning than that which is described by the market orthodoxy. The author is currently thinking through how to avoid the Mintzberg myth #9, around "rightly controlled by the public sector, for the sake of equity and economy" is best challenged, in the context of the correct and appropriate use of the private sector, to deliver additional capacity to assist with elective recovery. The pandemic has seen the overall approach to planning put centre-stage compared with the internal market alternative. Perhaps the implementation of the 2022 Act will deliver a revised structure of the NHS which is more reflective of the context of the time, which seemingly has seen a need for greater integration and the removal of market mechanisms.

7.4 Overall Conclusions

There is seemingly a changing mood around whether the NHS market approach is optimal and the practitioners in the finance part of the system seem less keen on its adoption even if they are struggling with the replacement. The

NHS finance epistemic community has not coalesced and galvanised around a common approach to the replacement which has probably meant the system has been in place for longer than it should have been. And the NHS finance epistemic community is somewhat uncertain as to whether they have a policy determination role.

The reasons for the longevity of the English NHS internal market policy are, in the views of the author, and his fellow practitioners, tested via the HFMA/PwC research and the HFMA Policy and Research Committee, are multiple in nature. Seemingly there was a collective acknowledgement that the internal market policy was failing along with the evidence to support that view, (which is described immediately below, referring to the 2012 Act). However, this was seemingly hard for politicians and practitioners to act upon, as they were unable to describe, agree on and then forge a different course. The inability to let go of the policy landscape which had been in situ since 1989, continues to be exceptionally hard, in terms of politics, policy embeddedness, the years of adoption, and consequent professional practice, as noted in Figure 7.1. The author believes that practitioners particularly struggle to acknowledge they need, to some extent, to topple the structures in which professionals inhabit, to develop a more integrated health and care approach. The author often describes, in his current role, the need to work more closely with local government colleagues and unlearn the muscle memory associated with internal market practices. At the centre of the current policy environment is a sentiment prevalent in a recent HFMA event reviewing the "ICBs after one year of their existence" which noted, "when you have seen how one ICB operates, you can conclude…how only one ICB operates". Meaning that each part of the health and care system is trying to individually, and collectively, chart a different and more collaborative course in health policy, following the 2022 Act. That course, however, is contingent on the local relationships and other factors. This makes local determination important, and therefore some elements of the national policy approach less relevant, in the view of the author.

Based on the answers to the research questions, the author concludes that the 2012 Act was the wrong set of reforms, and the internal market has remained a permanent fixture beyond the point at which there was a consensus for the need for a change of policy. The decade from 2012 to 2022, as well as being a very austere decade in terms of fiscal policy, could therefore also be described as a decade wasted in terms of the need for evidenced policy and a change in policy course for the English NHS. There was evidence from Market 2 of the problems within the system and the practical problem of getting an internal market in health to ever work. Whether or not these problems were due to (a) how the system was set up, (b) the failure of practitioners to implement it, or (c) the inability of the system or politicians to make tough choices at the point of market exit or failure, is contested. The author and the epistemic community he is part of would strongly advocate for a move away from the NHS internal market, based on:

- The conclusions of the House of Commons Select Committee report back in 2010. (Section 2.4)
- The view that the current payment system for health in the English system is probably rewarding the wrong things, in terms of a somewhat aged set of service and product definitions, which probably entrench the hospital sector's provider interest. (Section 4.2)
- The view is that the current NHS system and finance regime are not working well. It sees the financial problems of the English NHS residing predominantly in the provider hospital sector when the problem probably needs to reside in a series of local systems. These systems need to try and integrate health and care, to potentially avoid costly, and potentially unnecessary, hospital stays, via more integrated community and social care provision. (Section 4.3)
- The failed Failure Regime, which has not been utilised since two somewhat discredited attempts in 2012 and 2013, didn't manage to achieve an "exit" of inefficient provision. (Section 4.5)
- The author's senior finance practitioner experience, is associated with working in the NHS system at a regional and national level, and based on a Derbyshire level, trying to improve care for his local population and his own family. (Sections 5.1 and 6.3)
- The fact that there is a somewhat overwhelming finance practitioner belief that the current system is to a large extent broken and needs fundamental reform. (Section 5.2)
- The political consensus (via the 2015 and 2017 election manifestos), at least at a rhetorical level, is that care integration is the primary goal, and the internal market should not be allowed to get in the way of that goal (Section 6.2).

The evidence that the 2012 Act was the wrong set of reforms was not really challenged in real-time by the epistemic finance practitioner groups that were administering the NHS internal market. As the attitudinal research and Focus Group research shows, however, there was and still is a growing acknowledgement of the need to change, which eventually culminated in the 2022 Act. The HFMA, therefore, is working actively to try and promote an approach to NHS finance which exploits the benefits of the 2022 Act (HFMA 2023a, b and c). CIPFA is also trying to promote an approach to health and care integration (CIPFA, 2022) but it is also currently somewhat focused on the difficult state of local government finance itself. In the view of the author, the epistemic groups of NHS and public finance (both HFMA and CIPFA) tend to lag the politics and policy development phases of the NHS public policy and are not actively contributing to them in real-time. The author therefore considers that there is a role for practitioners in more directly influencing policy, but as we have often discussed both in the HFMA trustee and the CIPFA council meetings, it is difficult for these bodies, (as apolitical bodies, representing practice), to make statements which may be regarded as being overtly political, even though the policy landscape and the political processes are very well intertwined.

The author, and a number of his fellow ICB Directors of Finance/CFOs are currently spending much of their time with local government colleagues and GPs, trying to form conclusions on how we can better coordinate care for very high-risk individuals who may be presenting with healthcare problems which have at their root cause social, social-isolation and deprivation-related causation. We may therefore need to have a fundamentally different conversation about the role of the NHS where, how and whether we easily can effect changes to health and well-being and where those impacts best occur. We also need to have a conversation concerning the role of the state in the arena of the long-term care of the elderly versus the personal and family responsibility for that care. These root causes of disease conversations are taking place concurrently within a health system in which our ability to intervene in disease prevention and cure is growing at an accelerated rate. This is an articulation of the population and technology challenge (see Figure 1.1), articulated earlier, and these socially determined, chronic illness challenges need a different system design and architecture.

Without wishing to denigrate anyone working in the retail sector or the pivotally important role that GPs play in managing care at a local level, the best metaphor the author can muster in terms of the 2012 Act is "why would you entrust the corner shop keepers (again) to try and radically reform the super-markets and the super-market supply chain". The 2012 Act put GPs even more centre stage in the commissioning of health. The system then and now needs to address fundamental changes in how services are provided, and GPs may not be best placed to fulfil a broader policy role. GPs are part of the delivery mechanism of health, and they do not currently have the tools, or the time, to try and impactfully change the way we deliver care within the existing system. The majority of GPs, in the membership organisations, the CCGs, the last commissioning market incarnation, do not easily identify with the commissioning role or wish to undertake it, in the author's experience. GPs do wish to help to improve and better coordinate care, but there may be an alternative and more impactful mechanism to deliver this. Therefore 'Market

3˙ failed and was disbanded during the pandemic and the Health and Care Act (2022) replaced it with something different. We could take the Dorrell (in Stubbs (ed) (2018)) view of, "if at first you don't succeed try, try again", in respect of NHS commissioning, or we need to try and have a different conversation. The reality of the current English NHS is that it is having to define doing something different locally, to operate beyond the internal market, as the precise 'recipe' for the required change is unclear, despite the 2022 Act.

It should be stressed, that the author and a number of his ICB and wider finance colleague in the NHS finance community, do believe we need a good helping of healthy competition in healthcare delivery. The important point is what sort of competition we need. The author, and most people he has and does work with within his NHS England career, are quite well-motivated to try and ensure that they are delivering the best possible health and care system possible, that is both clinically and cost-effective. Not least because their own families and friends need that service routinely or at times of crisis, and we also pay taxes. What may be currently impeding some of that 'knightly' behaviour, could be the fragmented system we have generated to avoid 'knavishness'. If the internal market did have a New Public Management (NPM) policy origination to challenge bureaucracy and the bureaucrats within it. Then if the system adoption of the policy requires the 'street-level bureaucrats'/actors within the system to embrace the policy and implement it, logically, we have a policy approach doomed to failure. Namely, why would one trust the 'knaves' to appropriately challenge themselves, if they understood the policy and why would they be keen to correct their own 'knavish' behaviour? (Le Grand, 2003).

Of course, we need to be able to challenge the producer interest in healthcare supply, and the over-medicalisation of healthcare supply and many of the author's fellow NHS finance epistemic community understand that tension. The larger proportion of GDP spent in the US system, with potentially worse overall outcomes, could perhaps be explained by some elements of the supply side in the USA system being unchecked, as described by Scheider et al (2017). However, we all agree in the finance NHS community that we may need to be better coordinated in responding to that supply challenge; and we might need to concede that there is scope for public service and servant ethos, in the health and care system, that might be categorised by a wish akin Hippocratic Oath to "help the sick according to our own abilities and judgements, but never with a view to injury and wrongdoing". The finance epistemic community could have knightly aims that are worthy of exploration.

In his management career, the author would note that the approach to the management of staff can be slightly self-fulfilling. If staff are managed based on

(a) needing to curb the worst excesses of lazy and errant behaviour; as opposed to (b) trying to ensure everyone is delivering and is motivated to deliver the best they can; then via management approach (a) staff have a greater tendency to exhibit the very behaviour we would wish to avoid. Healthcare system and public policy management could reflect the author's micro, self-fulfilling prophecy, and personal management conclusion. Indeed, this negative view of public servants as displayed by New Public Management theorists, is not recognised by the author, and the consequence of treating them in this way generates the costs and disadvantages described by Seddon (2008).

In terms of the broader conclusions on the concept of policy persistence Kay (2005) the author would observe that the sheer complexity of the health and care system does lend itself to not trying to change the status quo too much for fear of unintended consequences. As the author keeps stating when trying to get coalitions, both in South Yorkshire, and nationally, to move their position on the disbenefits of the internal market and operate differently, as a consequence, he notes, "just because we understood how to operate in it (the NHS internal market), it didn't mean it was securing optimal outcomes". All agreeing (across the NHS finance and broader managerial community of practice) on the new "recipe" requires that common understanding and feel for how the new approach will operate at a local level and secure better results. The lack of potential agency that the epistemic public finance groups, that the author closely observes, (and is one of), in terms of both HFMA and CIPFA is understandable, perhaps, given the lack of a well-evidenced alternative to the current approach and an agreement on it. Also, the continued fractures between commissioning and provision, and between DHSC and DLUHC, despite the 2022 Act, continue to hamper an agreement on the revised approach, and there a confusion as to how much the act has reality changed things. As stated in section 2.2, perhaps the reason for the difficulty in implementing the internal market in health was the very same reason that it is now proving so difficult to dismantle.

> One general point is the effect of the bureaucratic and professional ownership within the state, which makes any attempt to reform policy a much longer process than was anticipated by neoliberal politicians. (Turner, 2008: 161)

7.5 Recommendations

There are three categories of recommendations associated with the research completed. Micro (related to NHS finance)

1. There is a pressing need for the NHS finance system to better understand

the wider needs and requirements of patients and citizens and operate beyond the boundaries of the existing statutory structures in health, to deliver improvements in health and wellbeing.

2. This requires a step-change in terms of ensuring services deliver good value as opposed to ensuring that individual organisations are delivering financial performance against relatively narrow financial criteria.

3. This will require an improved understanding of the different costs and approaches to the delivery of treatment and care and the improved development of descriptions of outcomes, and an approach to understanding overall costs of treatment and care which is less reliant on costing specific inputs using old historic activity definitions, such as those which are used for existing costing and pricing in the English NHS.

4. There needs to be greater convergence between the understanding of costs and the nature of services provided by local government, alongside the services delivered by the NHS, with closer co-operation between the two areas to improve healthy life expectancy for the most disadvantaged.

Meso (related to the English NHS)

5. The commissioning and provision split has not worked in the best interests of patients and a significant debate needs to take place to establish the best approach to utilising the existing management and clinical resources, within the English NHS, to best enable changes to improve the delivery of care.

6. The author recommends the blueprint of a tidied-up NHS, (Paton (2016) shown in Table 2.2, be adopted. This goes further than the 2022 Act and suggests further changes to the structures around provision. In addition, there should be a further debate on the centrality of GPs, in the delivery mechanism for health. The author would seek GP voices and participation in the management structure of the new integrated providers, and he would wish to see a fully inclusive GP arm of the integrated provider, under a single unified purchaser and provider statutory structure. This goes further than the 2022 Act and merges commissioning back with provision at an ICP level as a "Local NHS board".

7. The democratic oversight of the integrated "Local NHS Board" needs to be better aligned with the delivery of both health and care. Social care delivered via local government already has democratic accountability through local councillors. Although some respondents in the HFMA/

PwC research were keen to mandate a revised approach to delivery from the NHS centre, it is unlikely that there is a universal model for delivery available that will enable the response to the overall challenge of technology and the population needs. It is therefore suggested that the accountability for the new integrated "Local NHS Board" may better sit with the local population that it serves and a closer connection with local government may be preferable and less duplicative than the current oversight structures in the English NHS.

8. If these changes were adopted there would need to be a different conversation about the governance of providers, who are far more associated with tertiary and supra-regional work. At the moment, the pricing system probably does not reflect the costs of this care and it is possible that the grouping of the new "Local NHS Boards", linked to social and primary care, were less aligned to this more complex provision, which may need a different management, funding and governance model. Before the Griffiths Reforms, tertiary providers were managed differently to providers with close links to primary and community care. Something like this split between tertiary and secondary care, as currently happens in the Netherlands, (Jeurissen and Maarse 2021), may need to be revisited to best manage more specialist provision.

Macro (related to broader public policy)

9. Given the broad political consensus on the need to change the policy associated with the English NHS in 2017, there is a need to better establish an all-Party health public policy, to enable changes in structures, and approaches, where and when they are required. If all the parties want such a change, including the Secretary of State (when the HFMA/PwC report was discussed with him), but there was no time to deliver that change this does tell us something about the potential inefficiency of state provision.

10. There is probably also the need for greater clarity on the evaluation of policy, to ensure it meets the objectives that are laid down for it. The notion that the English NHS could not explain the costs of the purchaser/provider split, (as reported to the 2010 Health Select Committee), is understandable given the complexity of the system, but not entirely defensible.

11. There is also the need to overtly describe the complexity and ease with which policy is likely to be disseminated, at the outset, to better understand the level of clarity and simplicity with which that policy will be rolled out. In the context of the English NHS internal market, if the policy overtly

was to challenge the self-serving 'street-level bureaucrats', and the policy needed so much of their influence to enable adoption, that was unlikely to work, with hindsight.

7.6 Proposed Further Research

There are several areas of further research which are worthy of consideration in the context of this study. Some of these are already underway in the ongoing dissemination of this research and the author's wider role. Some are suggested as potential areas for improvement to the methodology used for this thesis and others are further areas of inquiry that could be suggested building on the broader conclusions reached. The author has written this thesis to try and contextualise the current NHS internal market and the competing accounts of its effectiveness and development. The author will be sharing drafts of this thesis with the research participants for feedback and would hope to publish a version of it, via the HFMA, to try and precipitate further debate, and to provide an example of doctoral-level study for finance and wider NHS, local government and wider public accountant practitioner colleagues.

Further action research and trying to influence current NHS financial policy and the internal market, is underway and will continue through the HFMA and CIPFA. The author continues to chair the Policy and Research Committee and continues in his role as a Trustee. Through this the author is currently engaged in two specific projects; one relates to the approach to stabilising the finance position of the provider sector, which was one of the recommendations in the HFMA/PwC report. The second relates to some joint work and HFMA on the improved engagement between health and local government to ensure that there is an improved and common approach to the joint oversight of health and care and an improved understanding between the two sectors. Also, the author has contributed to a recent publication from CIPFA on Integrating Care (2022) and is about to chair a panel on how the NHS and Local Government should work more closely together.

Following conversations with one of the Derbyshire MPs, who sits on the All-Party Parliamentary Heath Policy Working Group (APPG), the author has discussed the content of the initial PwC report on system architecture and the second HFMA/PwC report on changes to the finance regime. Now that a full draft of the thesis is available the author will discuss this further with local MPs. The direct engagement with the Health APPG, and the recommendations and areas covered within this report, could help with the vexatious issue of where policy change proposals can be suggested to try and improve the current NHS managerial and financial regime. This difficult issue was discussed extensively at the HFMA Policy and Research Committee and will be discussed further, prior to any such further step. The author would seek the backing on the best approach to influencing policy, with a mandate from the HFMA and CIPFA, to achieve the best results.

Recommendations were made on how to improve the secondary analysis of the statutory data in Chapter 4. Adopting the suggestions made around improving the commissioning to provision data mapping would be worthwhile.

Further research into stakeholder views on the internal market, such as different professional views on the existing system, mirroring the work done by HFMA/PwC on financial professionals would be desirable. The author would be keen to seek the views of the wider professions in health, using the approach in this report with other professions, doctors, nurses, allied health professionals and wider management within the system. The author continues to believe that the approval of the prevailing policy environment is a large determinant of some of the discretionary effort that employees in the system bring to work. It would be worthwhile therefore to both understand multi-disciplinary perspectives on the existing system and understand the consensus for any potential changes.

The author has also considered the approach to measuring attitudes to the existing internal market system within the leadership communities forming as part of the ICS process. Looking at those ICS participant attitudes may enable an approach to improved system alignment in ICSs, via an understanding of different stakeholder views. If different executives and stakeholders involved have aligned views on the role and approach to the internal market or the need for its replacement, this should lead to a more unified view on the role of the ICS, and improved performance of the local healthcare system. This understanding could be an interesting and valuable further line of inquiry.

The English NHS finance regime post-pandemic is also of interest and could be subject to further study. There have been approaches to try and incentivise elective work in both 2022/23 and 2023/24 called the Elective Recovery Fund. It is unclear the extent to which this PbR-type mechanism has been effective in helping reduce the elective backlog and the author has written (unsuccessfully) on trying to ensure this approach was not adopted. The author's claim has been the effects of the pandemic (on the workforce and other structural factors in the NHS) have impeded elective recovery (e.g. social care provision frailty), not the absence of a fee-for-service model for elective care itself. Through the policy of the Elective Recovery Fund, one can perhaps see an instance of how the old internal market policy and approach remains.

Penultimately, further work on the areas where top-down policy can be effective, or where there needs to be full stakeholder engagement in the co-design to enable successful public policy delivery and implementation, would be helpful. There are quasi-market parallels in education which would seem to be of interest. One could claim that the internal market in higher education seems somewhat embedded. The approach to parent and pupil choice in primary and secondary education seems a little more contentious. A comparative public policy analysis on the role of the four sectors; (i.e. primary education, secondary education, universities and health) and the potential importance and competing roles of (i) market structures, (ii) targets, (iii) fundamental system thinking, (iv) management improvements and (v) wider public policy initiatives, in each of these four sectors; is likely to give some further insight on where different policy types can have the biggest impact.

Finally, given the author's participation in comparative financial management work between Australia, the USA, The Netherlands and the UK, some work could be performed to look at the relative effectiveness of markets in healthcare from an international perspective. This could try and establish what may have made English NHS market policy better, and how it may have been supported by an improved approach to implementation, or by looking at the different approaches to care integration in different countries. This would help bring to light some of the contextual and wider factors that may lead to the success or failure of markets as a mechanism to deliver improvement in public policy, and whether an integrated alternative may be preferable.

REFERENCES

Abayomi, K., Gelman, A. and Levy, M. (2008) Diagnostics for Multivariate Imputations Journal of the Royal Statistical Society Applied Statististics 57, Part 3, pp. 273–291

Alderwick, H., Dunn, P., McKenna, H., Walsh, N., Ham, C. (2016) Sustainability and Transformation Plans in the NHS. London: Kings Fund

Allen, P., Checkland, K., Moran, V., Peckham S. (2020) Commissioning Healthcare in England: Evidence, Policy and Practice Bristol: Policy Press

Araral, E., Fritzen, S., Howlett, M., Ramesh, M., Wu, X. (Eds) (2013) Routledge Handbook of Public Policy. London: Routledge

Ashworth J. (ed.) (2018) A Picture of Health: The NHS at 70 and its future. London: Fabian Society

Baggot R. (2007) Understanding Health Policy. Bristol: Policy Press

Barber M. (2007) Instruction to Deliver: Fighting to Transform Britain's Public Services. London: Methuen

Berger, M.C. and Messer, J. (2002) Public financing of health expenditures, insurance, and health outcomes, Applied Economics, 34(17), pp. 2105-211

Barrett S. (2004) 'Implementation Studies: Time for a Revival? Personal reflections on 20 years of Implementation Studies', Public Administration, 82(2), pp.249-262

Berry W. and Sanders M. (2000) Understanding Multivariate Research: A Primer for Beginning Social Scientists. Boulder: Westview Press

Bevan G. And Hood C. (2006) 'What's Measured is What Matters: Targets and Gaming in the English Public Healthcare System', Public Administration, 84(6), pp.517-538

Bhaskar, R. (1978) A Realist Theory of Science (2nd Ed.). Hassocks: Harvester

Blaikie, N. (2007) Approaches to Social Enquiry (2nd Ed.). Cambridge: Polity

BMJ (2017); NHS in 2017: the long arm of government 356 doi: https://doi.org/10.1136/bmj.j41 (Published: 13 January 2017)

Blakemore, K. and Warwick-Booth, L. (2013) Social Policy: An Introduction (4th Ed.). New York: McGraw Hill

Bowling, A. (2009) Research Methods in Health: Investigating Health and Health Services. Milton Keynes: Open University Press

Bottery, M. and Wright, N. (2019) Writing a Watertight Thesis: A Guide to Successful Structure and Defence London: Bloomsbury

Brown, M. and Payne, S. (1990) Introduction to Social Administration in Britain. London: Routledge

Bruyn, S. (1963) The Methodology of Participant Observation, Human Organization, 22:3, Ithaca, New York: Society for Applied Anthropology

Bryman, A. and Burgess R. (1994) Analyzing Qualitative Data. London: Routledge

Burgess, H. Sieminski, S. Arthur, L. (2006) Achieving Your Doctorate in Education. London: Sage

Centre for Policy Studies (2018) A Royal Commission on the NHS: The Remit: https://cps.org.uk/research/a-royal-commission-on-the-nhs-the-remit/ (Accessed: October 2022)

CIPFA (2022) Integrating care: policy, principles and practice for places CIPFA

Coate, S. and Morris, S. (1999) 'Policy Persistence', The American Economic Review, 89(5), pp. 1327-1336

Cohen, L, Manion, L., Morrison, K. (2007) Research Methods in Education (sixth ed.). London: Routledge

Cooper Z., Gibbons S., Jones S. and McGuire A (2012) Does Competition Improve Public Hospitals Efficiency? Evidence from a Quasi-Experiment in the English NHS. Centre for Economic Performance Discussion Paper 1125

The Conservative Party (2015) The Conservative Party Manifesto: Strong Leadership, A Clear Economic Plan, A Brighter More Secure Future. London: The Conservative Party

The Conservative Party (2017) The Conservative Party Manifesto: FORWARD, TOGETHER: Our Plan for a Stronger Britain and a Prosperous Future. London: The Conservative Party

Creswell, J. (2009) Research Design: Qualitative, Quantitative and Mixed Methods Approaches. London: Sage

Crotty, M. (1998) The Foundations of Social Research: Meaning and Perspective in the Research Process. London: Sage

Department of Health (1989) Working for Patients, London: HMSO

Department of Health (2005) Creating a Patient-led NHS. London: HMSO

Department of Health (2007) Introduction of Payments by Results. London: DHSC

Department of Health (2011) Briefing Note on Government Amendments to Health and Social Care Bill: Report Stage (Commons) September 2011

Downs, A. (1957) 'An Economic Theory of Political Action in a Democracy', Journal of Political Economy, 65, pp. 135–150.

Drake, P. and Heath, L. (2011) Practitioner Research at Doctoral Level: Developing Coherent Research Methodologies. London: Routledge

Enthoven, A. (1985) Reflections on the management of the National Health Service: An American looks at incentives to efficiency in health services management in the UK. London: Nuffield Provincial Hospitals Trust

Exworthy, M., and Halford, S. (Eds.) (1999) Professionals and the New Managerialism in the Public Sector. Milton Keynes: Open University Press

Exworthy, M., Peckham, S., Powell, M. and Hann, A. (Eds.) (2012) Shaping Health Policy: Case Study Methods and Analysis. Bristol: Policy Press

Exworthy M., Mannion, R. and Powell, M. (Eds.) (2016) Dismantling the NHS?: Evaluating the Impact of Health Reforms. Bristol: Policy Press

Exworthy M., Mannion, R. and Powell, M. (Eds.) (2023) The NHS at 75: The State of UK Health Policy. Bristol: Policy Press

Ferlie, E., Ashburner, L., Fitzgerald, L., Pettigrew, A. (Eds.) (1996) The New Public Management in Action Oxford: The Oxford University Press

Fox, A. (2018) A New Health and Care System – Escaping the invisible asylum. Bristol: Policy Press

Giddens, A. (1998) The Third Way: The Renewal of Social Democracy. Cambridge: Polity Press

Glennerster, H. (1995) British Social Policy Since 1945. London: Blackwell

Gray, M. (2017) How to Get Better Healthcare (3rd Ed.). Oxford: Oxford University Press

Greener, I. (2002) 'Understanding NHS Reform: The Policy-Transfer, Social Learning, and Path-Dependency Perspectives', Governance, 15, pp.161-183

Greener, I. (2005) 'The Potential of Path Dependency in Political Studies', Politics, 25(1), pp.62-72

Greener, I., Harrington, B., Hunter, D., Mannion, R. and Powell, M. (2014) Reforming Healthcare: What's the evidence? Bristol: Policy Press

Greer, S. (2004) Territorial Politics and health policy: UK Health Policy in Comparative Perspective. Manchester: Manchester University Press

Griffiths, R. (1983) NHS Management Enquiry – Griffiths Report. London: DHSS

Guba, E.G. (1990) The Paradigm Dialogue. Newbury Park, CA: Sage

Gujarati, D. (1988) Basic Econometrics. New York: McGraw-Hill

Haeder, S.F. (2012) 'Beyond Path Dependence: Explaining Healthcare Reform and Its Consequences', Policy Studies Journal, 40(S1), 65-86

Harker, R. (2019) NHS funding and expenditure - Briefing Paper CBP0724. House of Commons Library

Ham, C. et al (2012) A Report to the Department of Health and NHS Future Forum: Integrated Care for Patients and Populations: Improving Outcomes by working together. London: King's Fund

Ham, C. (2009) Health Policy in Britain (6th Ed.). Basingstoke: Palgrave Macmillan

Hart, E. and Bond, M. (1995) Action Research for Health and Social Care: A Guide to Practice. Milton Keynes: Open University Press

Haas, P. (1992) 'Introduction: epistemic communities and international policy coordination', International Organization, 46(1), pp.1–35.

Hayek, F. (1944) The Road to Serfdom. London: Routledge

HFMA/PwC (2018) Making Money work in the health and care system. London: PwC

HFMA (2023 a)) System decision-making and governance HFMA

HFMA (2023 b)) Resources and funding to reduce health inequalities HFMA

HFMA (2023 c)) Professional development for finance staff at integrated care boards (ICBs) HFMA

Hicks, T. (2013) 'Partisan Strategy and Path Dependence: The Post-War Emergence of Health Systems in the UK and Sweden', Comparative Politics, 45(2), 207-226

Hill, M. and Hupe, P. (2002) Implementing Public Policy: Governance in Theory and in Practice. London: Sage

Hill, M. (2005) The Public Policy Process (4th Edition). London: Pearson

Hirschmann, A. (1969) Exit, Voice and Loyalty: Responses to the Decline in Firms, Organisations and States. Cambridge, Mass.: Harvard University Press

Hirschman, A. (1991) The Rhetoric of Reaction: Perversity, Futility, Jeopardy. Cambridge, Mass.: Harvard University Press

House of Commons (2011) Health and Social Care Bill Report Stage and Third Reading in House of Commons, 6th and 7th September 2011

House of Commons Health Select Committee (2010) Commissioning: Fourth Report of Session 2009/10. London: The Stationary Office

House of Commons Health Committee (2018) Integrated Care: organizations, partnerships and system - Seventh Report of Session 2017–19. London: The Stationary Office

House of Commons Treasury Committee (2011) Private Finance Initiative - Seventeenth Report of Session 2010–12. London: The Stationary Office

Jeurissen P. and Maarse H. (eds) (2021) The market reform in Dutch health care: Results, lessons and prospects European Observatory on Health Systems and Policies

John, P. (1998) Analysing Public Policy. London: Pinter

Kay, A. (2005) 'A Critique of the Use of Path Dependency in Policy Studies', Public Administration, 83, pp.553-571

Kvale, S., and Brinkmann, S. (2009) Interviews: Learning the craft of qualitative research interviewing, (2nd Ed.). Thousand Oaks, California: Sage

Kingdon, J.W. (1995) Agendas, Alternatives and Public Policy (2nd ed.). HarperCollins, New York.

King's Fund (2010) A High Performing NHS? A review of progress 1997 – 2010. London: The Kings' Fund

King's Fund (2011) Briefing – The Health and Social Care Bill Report and Third Reading 6-7 September 2011. London: The Kings Fund

Klein, R. (2013) The New Politics of the NHS (7th Edition). London: Routledge

The Labour Party (2015) The Labour Party Manifesto: Britain can be better. London: The Labour Party

The Labour Party (2017) The Labour Party Manifesto: For the many, not the few. London: The Labour Party

Lamb, S. (2012) The Health and Social Care Act 2012: A Handbook for NHS Foundation Trusts. Capsticks Solicitors LLP

Lansley, A. (2012) 'Competition is Critical for Reform', Health Service Journal, 16th February 2012

Le Grand, J. (1991) 'Quasi-Markets and Social Policy', The Economic Journal, 101(1), pp.256-267

Le Grand, J, Mays, N. and Dixon, J. (1998) Learning from the NHS Internal Market – A Review of the Evidence. London: King's Fund

Le Grand, J. (2003) Motivation, Agency and Public Policy: Of Knights & Knaves, Pawns & Queens. Oxford: Oxford University Press

Le Grand, J. (2007) The Other Invisible Hand: Delivering Public Services through Choice and Competition. Cambridge, Mass.: Princeton University Press

Leibenstein, H. (1966) 'Allocative Efficiency vs. X-Efficiency', American Economic Review, 56: pp.392–415

Letwin, O. (1988) Privatising the World: A Study of International Privatisation in Theory and Practice. London: Cassell

Leys, C. and Player, S. (2011) The Plot Against the NHS. London: Merlin Press

The Liberal Democrat Party (2015) The Liberal Democrat Party Manifesto: Stronger Economy, Fairer Society, Opportunity for Everyone. London: The Liberal Democrat Party

The Liberal Democrat Party (2017) The Liberal Democrat Party Manifesto: Change Britain's Future. London: The Liberal Democrat Party

The Liberal Democrat Party (2019) The Liberal Democrat Party Manifesto: Stop Brexit: Build a Brighter Future. London: The Liberal Democrat Party

Lincoln, Y.S. and Guba, E.G. (2000) Handbook of Qualitative Research. Thousand Oaks, CA: Sage

Lipsey, R. (1989) An Introduction to Positive Economics (7th Edition). London. Weidenfield and Nicolson

Lipsky, M. (2010) Street Level Bureaucracy: Dilemmas of the Individual in Public Services. New York: Russell Sage Foundation

Mannion, R., Davies, H., Marshall M. (2005) Cultures for Performance in Healthcare Milton Keynes: Open University Press

Marmot, M., Allen, J., Goldblatt, P., Boyce, T., McNeish, D. and Grady, M. (2010) The Marmot Review. London

Marmot, M., Allen, J., Boyce, T., Goldblatt, P., McNeish, D. and Morrison, J. (2020) Health Inequality in England: The Marmot Review 10 Years On. London: Institute of Health Equity

Marmor, T. (2007) Fads, Fallacies and Foolishness in Medical Care Management and Policy. Singapore: World Scientific Publishing

Matland, R. (1995) 'Synthesizing the Implementation Literature: The Ambiguity Conflict Model of Policy Implementation', Journal of Public Administration Research and Theory, 5(2), pp.145-174

Mays, N., Dixon, A. and Jones, L. (ed.) (2011) Understanding New Labour's market reforms of the English NHS. London: The King's Fund

May, P. and Winter, S. (2007) 'Politicians, Managers and Street Level Bureaucrats: Influences on Policy Implementation', Journal of Public Administration Research,19(3), pp.453 – 476

McConnell A. (2010) 'Policy Success, Policy Failure and Grey Areas In-Between', Journal of Public Policy, 30, pp.345-362

McGovern, L., Miller, G., Hughes-Cromwick, P. (2014) The Relative Contribution of Multiple Determinants of Health Outcomes. London: Health Affairs

McLoughlin, V. and Leatherman, S. (2003) 'Quality or financing: what drives design of the health care system?', BMJ Quality & Safety,12, pp.136-142.

McNiff, J., and Whitehead, J. (2003) You and Your Action Research Project (2nd Edition). London: Routledge

Mertens, D. M. (1998) Research Methods in Education and Psychology: Integrating Diversity with quantitative and qualitative approaches. Thousand Oaks, CA: Sage

Mintzberg, H. (2017) Managing the Myths of Healthcare: Bridging the gaps between care, cure, control and community. Oakland, Ca.: Berrett-Koehler

Monitor/NHSE (2013) A guide to the Market Forces Factor. London: Monitor/NHSE

Moran, M. (2002) 'Understanding the Regulatory State', British Journal of Political Science, 32(2), pp. 391-413

Morrell, K. (2006) 'Policy as Narrative: New Labour's reform of the National Health Service', Public Administration, 84(2), pp.367-385

National Audit Office (2012) Securing the future financial sustainability of the NHS. London: NAO

National Audit Office (2018) Sustainability and transformation in the NHS. London: NAO

Neuman, W. L. (2000) Social Research Methods: Qualitative and Quantitative Approaches (4th Edition). Boston: Allyn and Bacon

Niemietz, K. (2018) How to Structurally Reform the NHS to Improve Patient Outcomes. London: IEA

Niskanen, W. (1971) Bureaucracy and Representative Government. Chicago: Aldine Atherton

NHS (2019) The NHS long Term Plan. London: NHS

NHS (2019) The NHS's Recommendations to Government and Parliament for an NHS Bill. London: NHS

NHS Confederation (2011) Health and Social Care Bill – Briefing for Report Stage and Third Reading. London: NHS Confederation

Nuffield Trust (2021) Briefing: July 2021 - Second Reading of the Health and Care Bill. The London: Nuffield Trust

Office of Health Economics (2012) Competition in the NHS. London: Office of Health Economics

Outhwaite, L. (2012) The X-factor http://www.hfma.org.uk/blog/post/The-X-factor.aspx and Competitive Tension http://www.hfma.org.uk/blog/post/Competitive-Tension.aspx (Accessed: 24th Feb 2012)

Outhwaite, L. (2020) A financial framework to support system working, Healthcare Financial Management Association Available from: https://www.hfma.org.uk/news/blogs/blog-post/a-financial-framework-to-support-system-working (Accessed: 6 December 2020)

Papanicolas, I. and Smith, P. (eds.) (2013) Health System Performance Comparison: An Agenda for Policy, Information and Research. New York: McGraw Hill

Paton, C. (1998) Competition and Planning in the NHS (2nd Edition). Cheltenham: Stanley Thorns

Paton, C. (2006) New Labour's State of Health: Political Economy, Public Policy and the NHS. Aldershot: Ashgate

Paton, C. (2016) The Politics of Health Policy Reforms in the UK – England's Permanent Revolution. Basingstoke: Palgrave Macmillan

Pierson, P. (2000) 'Increasing Returns, Path Dependence, and the Study of Politics', American Political Science Review, 94(2), pp.251-267

Pollock, A. (2004) NHS PLC: The Privatisation of Our Health Care. London: Verso

Pollock, A., Macfarlane, A. and Greener, I. (2012) 'Bad Science concerning NHS competition is being used to support the controversial Health and Social Care Bill', LSE Academic Blog: https://blogs.lse.ac.uk/politicsandpolicy/bad-science-nhs-competition/ posted 5th March 2012

Porter, M.E. and Teisberg, E.O (2006) Redefining Healthcare: Creating Value-Based Competition Based on Results. Cambridge, Mass: Harvard Business School Press

Pressman, J. and Wildavsky, A. (1973) Implementation. Berkley: University of California Press

PwC (2016) Redrawing the health and social care architecture: Exploring the role of national bodies in enabling and supporting the delivery of local health and care services. London: PwC

Ranade, W. (ed.) (1998) Markets and Healthcare: A Comparative Analysis. London: Longman

Ross, F. (2007) 'Questioning path dependence theory: the case of the British NHS', Policy & Politics, 35(4), pp.591-610

Sabatier, P. and Mazmanian, D. (1983) The Implementation of Public Policy: A Framework of Analysis   US Institute of Government Affairs

Sabatier, P. (1986) 'Top Down and Bottom Up Approaches to Implementation Research: A Critical Analysis and Suggested Synthesis', Journal of Public Policy, 6(1), pp.21-48

Sackett, D.L., Rosenberg W.M., Gray, J.A., et al . (1996) 'Evidence based medicine: what it is and what it isn't', BMJ, 312(71)–doi:10.1136/bmj.312.7023.71

Saldin, R.P. (2017) When Bad Policy Makes Good Politics: Running the Numbers on Health Reform. Oxford: Oxford University Press

Schneider, E., Sarnak, D., Squires, D., Shah, A. and Doty, M. (2017) Mirror 2017: International Comparison Reflects Flaws and Opportunities for Better U.S. Health Care (Commonwealth Fund, July 2017). https://doi.org/10.26099/0mh5-a632

Schofield, J. and Sausman, C. (2004) 'Symposium on Implementing Public Policy: Learning from Theory and Practice', Public Administration, 82, pp.235- 248

Schon, D. (1983) The Reflective Practitioner: How Professionals Think in Action. New York: Basic Books

Seddon, J. (2008) Systems Thinking in the Public Sector: the failure of the reform regime and a manifesto for a better way. Charmouth: Triarchy Press

Sheaff., R (1991) Marketing for Health Services. Milton Keynes: Open University Press

Sheaff., R and Peel V. (1995) Managing Health Service Information Systems Milton Keynes: Open University Press

Sheaff., R (2002) Responsive Healthcare: Marketing for a Public Service Milton Keynes: Open University Press

Smith, J., Walshe, K. and Hunter, D. (2001) 'The "Redisorganisation" Of The NHS: Another Reorganisation Involving Unhappy Managers Can Only Worsen the Service', British Medical Journal, 323(7324), pp.1262-1263

Stoker, G. (1995) 'Intergovernmental relations', Public Administration, 73(1), pp.101-122

Silverman, D. (2011) Qualitative Research. London: Sage

Sirigari A. K. (2020) A Complete Model Diagnostics of Multivariate Linear Regression accessed via www.medium.com on 6th May 2024

Stacey, R. (1993) Strategic Management and Organisational Dynamics (4th ed.). London: Pitman

Stringer, E. (2007) Action Research. London: Sage

Stubbs, E. (ed.) (2018) The Health of the Nation: Averting the demise of universal healthcare. London:Civitas

Timmins, N. (2012) Never Again? – The Story of the Health and Care Act of 2012. London: King's Fund

Timmins, N. (2010) 'Healthcare on the brink of a cultural revolution', The Financial Times, 17th January 2010

Torfing, J. (2009) 'Rethinking path dependence in public policy research', Critical Policy Studies, 3(1), pp.70-83

Travis A. (2016) 'Thatcher pushed for breakup of welfare state despite NHS pledge' The Guardian, 25th November 2016 (accessed 10th April 2020): https://www.theguardian.com/politics/2016/nov/25/margaret-thatcher-pushed-for-breakup-of-welfare-state-despite-nhs-pledge

Trust Special Administrator of Mid Staffordshire NHS Foundation Trust (2012) Trust Special Administrators' - The main report. Presented to Parliament pursuant to s.65I of the National Health Service Act 2006

Trust Special Administrator - Appointed to the South London Healthcare NHS Trust (2013) Securing sustainable NHS services: the Trust Special Administrator's report on South London Healthcare NHS Trust and the NHS in south east London. Presented to Parliament pursuant to section 65I of the National Health Service Act 2006

Tuohy, C.H., Flood, C.M. and Stabile, M. (2004) 'How Does Private Finance Affect Public Health Care Systems? Marshaling the Evidence from OECD Nations', Journal of Health Politics, Policy and Law, 29(3), pp.359-396

Tullock, G., Seldon, A. and Brady, G.L. (2000) Government: Whose Obedient Servant. London: Institute of Economic Affairs

Tuohy, C. (1999) Accidental Logics: The dynamics of Change in the Health Care Arena in the United States, Britain and Canada. Oxford: Oxford University Press

Turner, R.S. (2008) Neo-Liberal Ideology: History, Concepts and Policy. Edinburgh: Edinburgh University Press

Walsh, K., Deakin, N., Smith, P., Spurgeon P., Thomas N. (1997) Contracting for Change: Contracts in Health, Social Care and Other Local Government Services. Oxford: Oxford University Press

Wenger, E. (1998) Communities of Practice: Learning, Meaning, and Identity. Cambridge University Press

Wickham-Jones, M. (1996) Economic Strategy and the Labour Party: Politics and Policy-Making 1970 to 1983. Basingstoke: MacMillan

Wildavsky, A. (1992) The New Politics of the Budgetary Process (2nd Edition). London: Harper Collins

Wilkinson, D. (2000) The Researcher's Toolkit: A Complete Guide to Practitioner Research. London: Routledge Falmer

Printed in Great Britain
by Amazon

52751668R00136